LOSE YOUR BELLY FOR GOOD!

by Jon Lipsey and Joe Warner

Managing Editor Chris Miller
Art Editor Ian Ferguson
Photography Glen Burrows
Model Leon @ WModels
Additional Photography iStock

Publisher Steven O'Hara
Publishing Director Dan Savage
Marketing Manager Charlotte Park
Commercial Director Nigel Hole

Printed by William Gibbons and Sons, Wolverhampton

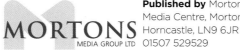

Published by Mortons Media Group Ltd,
Media Centre, Morton Way,
Horncastle, LN9 6JR
01507 529529

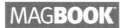

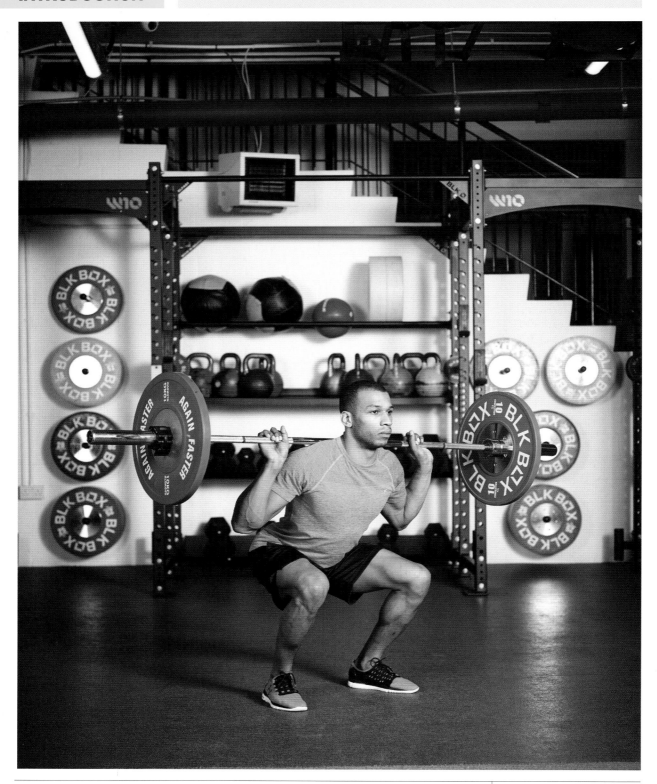

CONTENTS

006

Introduction

Learn everything you need to know about how the plan works as well as how you can eat and use supplements to build your best ever body.

026

Phase 1

Involves circuit-based sessions where your work rate is high and rest periods are short. This is designed to burn off fat and get you primed for Phase 2.

094

Phase 2

The workouts shift to focus more on building muscle so that you don't just burn off body fat but you also sculpt a lean and strong-looking physique

FAT LOSS LIES

Why most fat loss advice should be ignored, and what you should listen to

If you ask ten people how to lose body fat they will all give you an answer. The problem is that you'll get ten different answers. There are a couple of reasons for this. The first is that there is a lot of poor information out there about healthy and effective ways to improve your body composition. Fitness and fat loss is big business and that means there are a lot of people who want to make a quick buck off the back of dodgy fat loss promises. Whether it's a miracle pill, plan or powder, the chances are that the creator is more concerned with the thickness of their wallet than they are with the thinness of your waistline.

As a result, it's difficult to know who to listen to. It is, however, worth noting that when you get ten different views on how to eat and exercise it doesn't mean that at least nine of them are wrong. This is because there isn't just one approach that works although you need to appreciate that some are more useful than others. For example, there are things you can do that will be incredibly effective over a short period of time but are also unsustainable or unenjoyable. You might start an extreme plan and see good results initially but after a few weeks you'll run out of energy and motivation and you'll slip back to where you started or, worse, end up heavier and unhappier than when you started. You could also follow an approach that is effective but incredibly slow. That may be valid but we understand that you probably want to see results at a decent speed. The ideal plan, therefore, is one that is healthy, enjoyable and sustainable and that's what we aimed for when we created this eight-week programme.

PLAN FOR PROGRESS

This is an eight week plan because that's a good period of time during which you can make positive progress. The plan revolves around combining resistance training workouts and a smart approach to nutrition. The workout plan is split into two phases. Phase one involves doing circuit-based sessions where your work rate is high and rest periods are short. In phase two the workouts shift to focus more on muscle building so that you don't just burn off body fat but you also build a lean and strong-looking physique too. The nutrition plan includes plenty of protein, healthy fats and complex carbohydrates that are generally timed to be eaten around your workouts. Follow it and we're sure you'll be happy with the results. You'll also have a confident new answer to give if anyone ever asks you about the best way to lose fat.

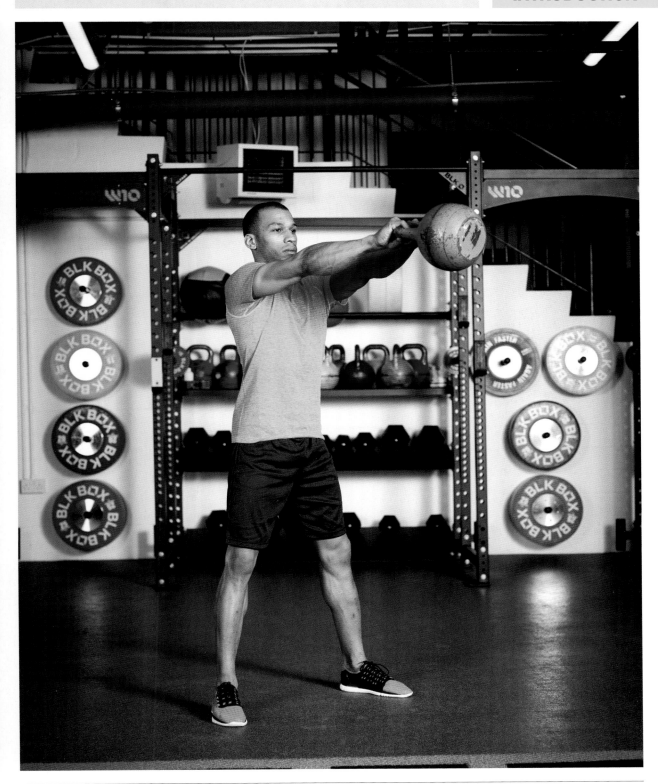

TRAIN FOR FAT LOSS

Discover the best way to exercise if you want to burn fat

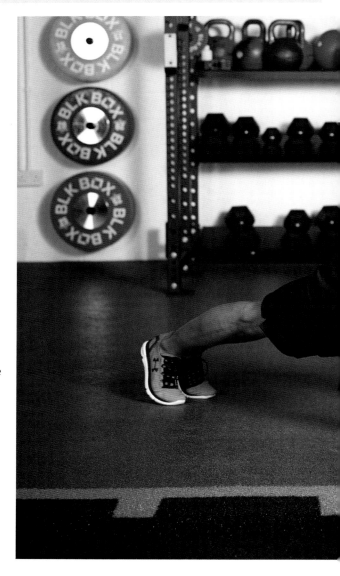

If you thought the best way to burn off excess body fat was to go for regular long-distance runs at a steady pace, it's time to think again. For years people have mistakenly believed steady-state cardio endurance exercise is the most effective method for losing weight. In fact, regularly performing such long, slow sessions – whether of running, rowing, cycling or swimming – isn't the right way to get slimmer.

GET INTENSE

The best method of torching body fat is to perform weight training sessions at a high intensity. Working out in this way will have a positive impact on your levels of testosterone – the male sex hormone responsible for a host of functions ranging from increased libido to higher muscle and lower body-fat levels. Levels of human growth hormone are also heightened after weight-training workouts, which instructs your body to burn fat and build new muscle tissue.

High intensity weight training also significantly works your cardiovascular system. Increasing the rate at which your heart and lungs have to work to pump blood, oxygen and other nutrients around your body has a positive effect on reducing body-fat levels.

DEBT PAID

During intense periods of exercise your lungs can't take in enough oxygen to provide your body with what it needs. This has the effect of creating an 'oxygen debt' within your body.

Just like any debt, this deficit needs to be repaid. Your body does this by increasing the amount of oxygen it consumes in the hours after your exercise session has finished. This phenomenon is known as excess post-exercise oxygen consumption, or EPOC, and this period of increased oxygen intake also increases the rate at which you burn calories, which will have a positive effect on your body composition.

Another benefit of any form of high-intensity exercise is that it causes lactic acid to accumulate in your muscle cells. While this build-up is responsible for the unpleasant feelings of 'muscle burn', elevated levels of this compound – which is a by-product of glucose metabolism – are thought to lead to an increase in the release of fat-torching growth hormones in the hours following your workout.

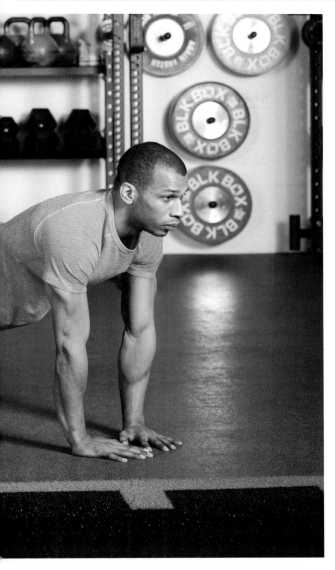

REST ASSURED

While lifting weights is one of the best ways to burn fat, simply picking up a heavy bar once and then walking away isn't the right approach to take. Yes, doing so will eventually make you stronger, but it will have very little effect on your body-fat levels.

You need to lift weights in a specific way to elicit the desired fat-burning response. For this programme that means you need to approach your three weekly weight training sessions in a particular way. You need to work hard for a set period of time and then take a short rest before lifting again.

Never giving your body enough time to recover is critical to whether your efforts to burn fat will be successful or

not. This technique, which really pushes you out of your comfort zone, is known as 'accumulated fatigue' and results in the maximum number of muscle fibres being broken down. It's also responsible for elevating lactic acid in your muscles and forcing your heart and lungs to work really hard. These factors combine to increase lean muscle mass and reduce fat stores to give you a better body.

That's why the workouts in the first four weeks of this plan are circuits, where you do one set of each exercise before resting. Taking very little rest between each individual exercise keeps your heart rate high and does the maximum amount of damage to your muscles, so it's vital you stick to the rest periods detailed in each workout. The longer you rest between the exercises, the less effective the workout will be and the less likely you are to get the results you want. Once you get more familiar with lifting weights the workout structure changes and you perform a mixture of supersets (where you do two exercises back to back without rest) and tri-sets (where you do three exercises back to back without resting).

THE LAST WORD

Even if you do everything right in the gym and perform the workouts perfectly, you'll still fall short of making positive changes to the way you look if you don't follow this programme's nutrition advice. It may be an old fitness cliché, but like all clichés it's based on more than a little truth: you can't out-train a bad diet. Turn to p16 to understand how the eight-week nutrition plan works and gain all the information you need to succeed.

WORKOUT BASICS

Simple answers to the most common training questions

Q I've tried and failed to lose weight in the past. Why will it work now?
If your previous efforts have been unsuccessful it has nothing to do with your body being resistant to exercise and everything to do with your approach. In other words, you probably didn't have a realistic goal, a focused and progressive training plan or eat the right foods at the right time. Anyone can lose body fat to transform significantly the way they look but that won't happen overnight. But the eight-week training and nutrition plan in this book, if followed without fault, will give you a better body.

Q Can I turn fat into muscle?
No, fat and muscle are two totally different types of tissue and it's impossible to turn one into the other. Muscle is active tissue that burns calories (and that's one of the reasons why it's useful to build muscle while simultaneously burning fat), while fat tissue stores excess energy. The right training programme will burn off these fat stores and build new muscle tissue, giving the appearance that one has turned into the other, but that isn't the case.

Q How many times a week do I need train?
This programme requires you to work out three times a week. You should aim to leave at least one day's rest between the weights sessions to give your body time to recover.

Q How closely do I need to follow the workout plan?
The closer you follow the plan, the better your results will be. Every workout has been designed to elicit a fat-burning response and forms an important part of a structured and progressive training plan that will significantly reduce the amount of fat you carry. Do the workouts in order for the best results possible.

Q What about sticking to the sets, reps and rest numbers detailed?
These are crucial too. You need to complete all the sets and reps while sticking to the rest periods between the moves. Failure to do so will limit the success of your fat-loss journey.

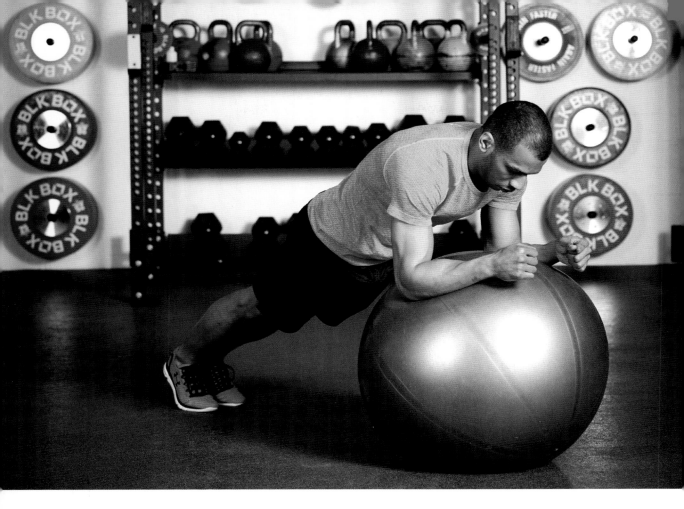

Q What if I can't complete all the sets and reps?
If this is the case, the weight you're lifting is too heavy and you need to reduce it. This programme isn't about lifting the heaviest weight possible, but exposing your muscles and cardiovascular system to the right amount of stress to make your body take positive steps towards becoming fitter and leaner.

Q How do I know which weights to use?
At first there will be a little bit of trial and error because the amount of weight you should be lifting will depend on a number of factors unique to you, such as age and training experience. It's always best to choose a light weight if you are unsure and stick to the reps at the right tempo. If you can complete the set with ease, you should increase the weight next time.

Q What should I do if my gym doesn't have the equipment used in some of the exercises in this plan?
This programme has been designed to be as easy and

efficient to follow as possible, with many moves in each of the circuits and supersets using the same piece of equipment so you don't waste time moving around the gym between moves. However, depending on the quality of your gym, some may not have exactly every single bit of kit you need. That's not a problem: just swap those moves for ones that target the same muscles which you can do with the equipment available to you.

Q Why do I need to do a Fat-Loss Finisher at the end of some of the weight-training sessions?
All three weight-training sessions each week are designed to build lean muscle mass and reduce body fat to radically transform your physique so that you look stronger and leaner. The Fat-Loss Finisher at the end of some sessions is designed to push your body even further out of its comfort zone to elicit the best fat-burning response possible by increasing the oxygen debt your body needs to repay and resulting in the right hormonal response to encourage the building of new muscle and the burning of fat cells.

LOSE YOUR BELLY FOR GOOD!

BIGGER AND STRONGER

The simple science behind adding muscle mass

Your body is a clever old thing. The process of muscle growth is essentially your body's response to the stress of weight training. It thinks, 'That was hard. I'd better do something about it so it's not as difficult next time.' When you perform resistance exercises, microscopic tears occur in your muscles. Your body responds to this 'microtrauma' by overcompensating: the damaged tissue is repaired and more is added, making your muscles bigger and stronger so the risk of future damage is minimised. This also means over time you need to increase steadily the weight you lift, because your muscles quickly adapt to deal with the stress. It's thought this damage to your muscle fibres is the reason for delayed onset muscle soreness, or DOMS, the symptoms of which include muscle soreness and stiffness in the days after a tough workout. That's why you should leave at least 48 hours between sessions that target the same muscle group. If you train those muscles again before they've had time to repair and rebuild you risk overtraining, which can result in reduced gains and injury.

48
The amount of time in hours you should ideally leave between training sessions focusing on the same muscle group

ANATOMY OF A MUSCLE

Muscles are made up of bundles of fibres contained in protective sheaths called fascia, which are then themselves bundled together. The biggest bundle is the muscle itself. Next are the fascicles, which contain muscle fibres. These are then divided into myofibrils, which are divided into myofilaments, made up from chains of sarcomeres.

1 TENDON Strong, connective tissue connecting muscle to bone.

2 EPIMYSIUM A layer of connective tissue encasing the entire muscle.

3 ENDOMYSIUM Connective tissue covering the muscle fibres. Also contains capillaries (tiny blood vessels) and nerves.

4 PERIMYSIUM A layer of connective tissue that bundles individual muscle fibres to create fascicles.

5 FASCICLE A bundle of individual muscle fibres.

6 MYOFILAMENTS These are the smallest fibre bundles, made up of sarcomeres, the basic unit of a muscle.

7 MUSCLE FIBRE Individual muscle fibres come in two main types: type 1 or slow-twitch, suited to endurance because they are slow to fatigue; and type 2 or fast-twitch, which are quick to fatigue and suited to fast movements.

HOW MUSCLES GROW

 1 WARM-UP
As your heart rate increases, blood is pumped into your muscles, warming them up and allowing them to extend fully. The blood also supplies the muscle fibres with oxygen. At the start of a rep, your muscles are under tension and stretched. As a result more blood is pumped into the protective sheaths of the muscle fibres, supplying even more oxygen and nutrients.

 2 SPARK
As you lift a weight, your central nervous system relays this to the nerves in the sheaths around the muscle fibres, telling the fibres to contract. If you do the exercise correctly your muscles will activate in a particular sequence, which your nervous system adapts to. As you repeat the workout, your nerves get more efficient, allowing you to do more. This is the first adaptation caused by weightlifting.

 3 CHEMICAL REACTION
Adenosine triphosphate (ATP) is the immediate energy source for these muscle contractions. It is broken down within the body's cells to release energy. The cells' creatine, phosphate and glycogen reserves are also converted into ATP. This process creates lactic acid as a by-product.

 4 THE BURN
Once the glycogen stores in your cells have been depleted and lactic acid starts to build up the muscle can't work efficiently, so you have to rest. As you do so, aerobic (oxygen-based) muscle respiration occurs, processing the lactic acid back into glycogen and giving you an energy source for the next set.

 5 SUCCESSFUL FAILURE
As you reach failure on the last set of a given exercise, your fast-twitch muscle fibres are completely fatigued. Microscopic tears ('microtears') occur in the myofilaments, the smallest fibre bundles in your muscles.

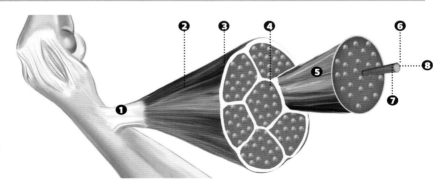 **6 REPAIR AND GROW**
Your muscles start to grow during the post-workout repair process. Your body fixes the microtears by adding the amino acids actin and myosin to the myofilaments, which also causes them to grow. Your muscles adapt to store more glycogen too, so there's more energy for the next workout. This also has the happy side effect of making the muscles slightly bigger.

8 BLOOD VESSEL Part of the body's circulatory system, blood vessels come in three types: arteries, responsible for transporting oxygenated blood away from the heart to the organs and tissues; capillaries, which enable the exchange of nutrients and waste products between the blood and tissues; and veins, which transport deoxygenated blood from the capillaries back to the heart.

GLOSSARY
Explanations of some common workout terms

COMPOUND LIFT
An exercise involving movement in two or more joints, such as the squat (hip and knee) and shoulder press (shoulder and elbow). Such lifts should form the basis of all programmes where increasing muscle size and strength are the aims because they recruit more of the muscle fibres responsible for those attributes.

FAILURE
When you're unable to lift the weight with correct form on the final rep of your set. This shocks your muscles into growing back bigger and stronger.

TRI-SETS
Three moves done back to back with little or no rest between them. They allow you to train with more volume in a shorter period.

HYPERTROPHY
Greek for 'excess nourishment', hypertrophy is an increase in the volume of a muscle or organ caused by enlargement of its cells.

ISOLATION LIFT
An exercise involving movement in only one joint, such as the biceps curl (elbow) and leg extension (knee). They're great at the end of a workout when you can work a muscle to failure.

MUSCLE PUMP
When muscles are engorged with blood after you've repeatedly shortened and lengthened it. Typically this occurs after weight training.

REPS
Abbreviation of repetition. One rep is the completion of a given exercise from start to finish through a full range of motion. The number of reps per set can vary from one to more than 20, depending on your goals.

REST INTERVAL
The time you take between exercises and/or sets, during which your muscles can replenish their energy stores. The amount of rest can be manipulated depending on your training goals.

SETS
A given number of reps of a single exercise performed consecutively without rest. The number of sets performed of each exercise can vary depending on the workout.

SUPERCOMPENSATION
The period after training and recovery when you're fitter and stronger than before. Training in this window will result in further gains in strength, size and fitness. Training before this window, on the other hand, can result in overtraining, while training after it has closed reduces your ability to make additional gains.

TEMPO
The speed at which you perform a lift. Tempo is detailed by a four-digit code, such as 4010. The first number is the time in seconds the weight is lowered; the second is the time in seconds the move is held at the bottom position; the third is the time in seconds that the weight it lifted (if 'X' is shown this means lift explosively); and the final digit is the time in seconds the weight is held at the top of the move.

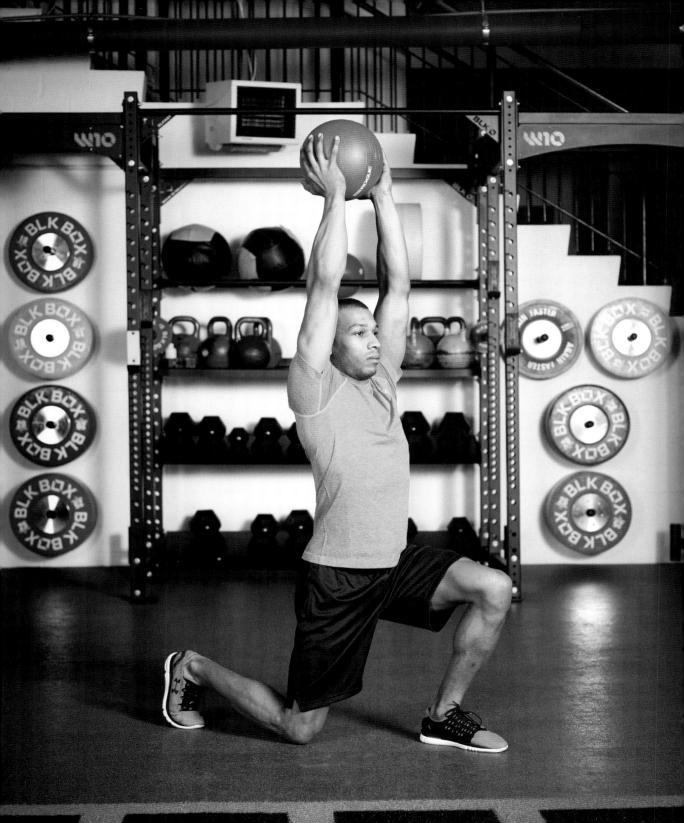

FOOD RULES

The principles behind your eight-week fat-loss nutrition plan

What you eat and when is critical for building a leaner body, which is why we have made following the eight-week nutrition plan in this book as easy as possible. At the start of each weekly chapter there is a seven-day meal plan for you to follow. To ensure you stick to the schedule, look at week one before you start and fill your cupboards, fridge and freezer with all the foods you'll need that week. Not having the right foods to hand will make it impossible to stick to the plan and have you reaching for the takeaway menus. These are the priciples upon which the nutrition plans are based.

PROTEIN FOR BREAKFAST...
Eating protein for breakfast is one the best things you can do when wanting to lose weight. Protein allows for a slow and steady rise in blood sugar levels, which keeps you feeling fuller for longer so you aren't tempted to reach for sweets to boost energy by mid-morning. It also helps repair the damage done to your muscles through training, and improves focus so you are more determined to stick to the diet plan throughout the rest of the day.

... AND PROTEIN WITH EVERY MEAL
People on a high-protein diet find it easier to lose weight, and it's hard to eat too much. Almost every meal in each plan contains a source of lean protein to ensure you get enough each day to repair your muscles, while burning fat.

PLENTY OF FRESH VEGETABLES
Along with protein, vegetables should form a significant part of each meal – roughly half, in fact. Veg is high in antioxidants and many essential vitamins and minerals to keep you fighting fit, and full of fibre, which will also help you feel full long after eating. Vegetables are also very low in calories.

CARBS AROUND TRAINING
Most of the carbs in the meal plans are to be eaten around your workouts. This is because carbs allow you to recover from training faster, and it's important you are fully energised for each session so you can push yourself. All these carbs rank low on the glycaemic index, which means they don't raise blood sugar levels too rapidly so your body is constantly in the best state to burn fat.

PLENTY OF WATER
Dehydration leads to poor focus and lack of motivation. These things can cause you to make poor food choices and perform badly in the gym, so aim to drink two to three litres a day, and more on training days. Water also flushes toxins and waste from your body, making you more efficient and helping you get fitter and leaner.

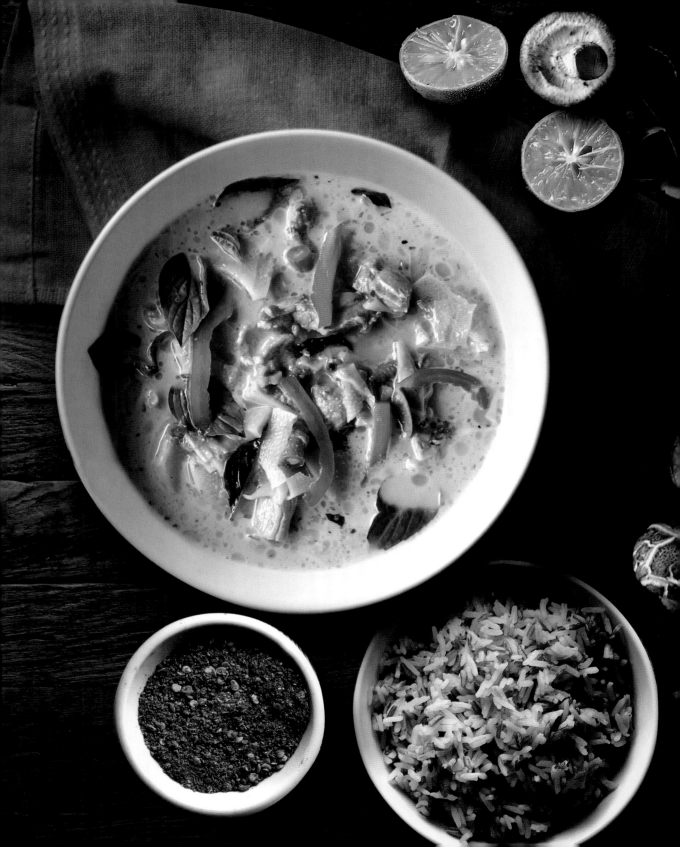

DIET BASICS
Discover the answers to common questions about this meal plan

Q How closely do I need to follow the weekly meal plans?
You need to follow them as closely as possible. Each meal plan has been designed to provide you with just the right amount of nutrients to allow your body to recover from training so you can attack the next session at 100%, without giving you any more than is necessary. Failing to stick to the key principles behind each day's diet will undo much of the hard work you put in at the gym.

Q Some of the meals aren't exactly exciting my tastebuds. Is there anything I do about that?
The majority of your meals over the next eight weeks will be based around lean sources of protein and fresh vegetables. What's not to like? If this is a radical departure from your normal diet, this is a good thing because you are likely to see results faster.

You need to remember that for the next eight weeks you are eating for a better body, not your tastebuds, so try to enjoy the new diet plan because it will make you leaner. If you do find the meals too bland to stomach, you can add spices, chilli flakes, garlic and herbs to give them some flavour and kick.

Q I find that I'm often hungry before I go to bed. Is this OK?
It may be that you experience a few more hunger pangs than you're used to when eating to lose weight, but this isn't necessarily a bad thing. It may simply be because your body is used to being fed more often and with foods that you now need to limit.

This programme's weekly meal plans have been designed to provide the right amount of protein and fat each day so you have enough energy to train hard and recover fully without leaving you hungry, because any more food than is necessary could be stored as fat. If you find you're hungry a lot of the time, you can increase the amount of meat and veg you eat, especially in the evenings.

Q How can I make sure I stick to the meal plans?
Organisation is key. You need to know what you're eating and when for the following seven days so you have all the supplies in your home and ready to eat. If you don't have what you need at hand, you're far more likely to stray from the plan and eat convenience foods that are high in carbs, especially sugar. Whenever possible, spend some time each evening preparing the next day's meals and snacks – that's one of the best ways to stay on the right path.

Q How can I reduce the cost of my weekly shopping?
Vegetables are inexpensive, but lean meat can be pricey. However, buying in bulk can significantly reduce your expenditure on food and is easy to do on this plan because all your meals for the next eight weeks are mapped out for you. Another advantage of shopping this way is you can batch cook and freeze meals for later in the programme.

Q Can I drink alcohol over the next eight weeks?
If you want to achieve the best results possible, you should steer clear of alcohol. There are many reasons for this. Alcohol is just empty calories – it contains energy but very few nutrients. Your body prioritises processing alcohol over other things, such as burning fat and building muscle. You're less likely to stick to your diet plan when under the influence of alcohol because it affects blood sugar levels and stimulates your appetite. It can be so tempting to skip the next day's training session if you're hungover.

If you can't avoid alcohol entirely, stick to the very occasional glass of red wine, but remember that every drink you have will limit the extent of your transformation.

Q How important are supplements to my progress?
Not as important as sticking to the meal plans. Supplements are just that - they supplement a varied and well-balanced diet to help you on your way to a better body. Some supplements, such as whey protein and omega 3 fatty acids, are more important than others when fat loss is your primary objective. For our full round-up of which supplements you may need and when best to take them, turn the page.

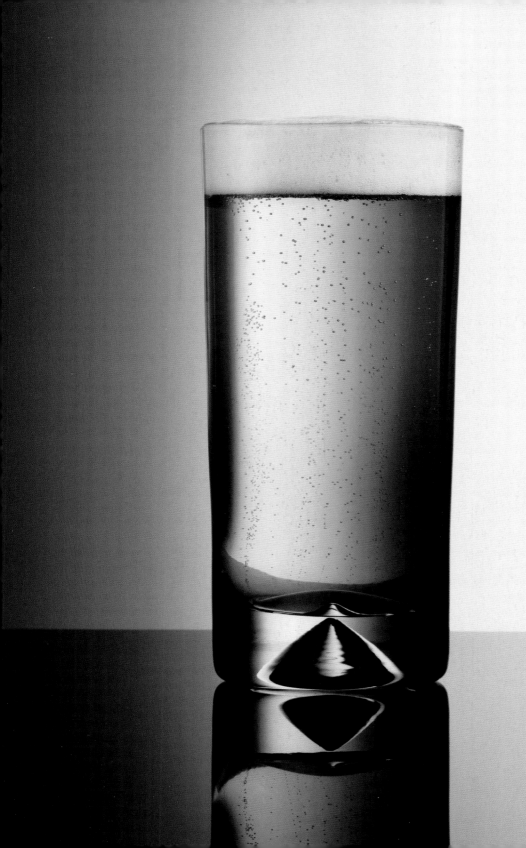

SUPER SUPPS

Take the right supplements at the right time for greater gains

Whether you regularly pack a protein shake in your gym bag or just chug the occasional isotonic sports drink, chances are you've used supplements at one time or another. The trouble is, the whole process can get a bit confusing – with every supplier claiming its brand is better filtered, or more efficient, or will pack on more muscle – to the point where you feel as if you need a degree in chemistry to understand what you're putting into your body. Don't worry, help is at hand. The science behind some supplements may be slightly baffling, but over the next few pages we've put together the definitive guide to the latest developments in supplement science: what you need, when you need it, why you need it and what – if any – are its potential pitfalls. It's possible you'll find something to send your training gains through the roof, or you might just learn a bit more about the stuff you're already using. Either way, next time you put in a hard day at the gym, you'll know you're getting the nutritional back-up you need.

WHAT SUPP?
We answer the most frequently asked supplement questions

Q Can I get all the nutrition I need from my daily diet?
Yes, if you really watch what you eat. Having said that, you may find that sometimes getting the optimum amount of certain substances for your training means eating a lot. For example, consuming the amount of creatine many trainers recommend would mean eating an awful lot of beef, which would not be feasible in most cases. Use supplements to fill the gaps in your diet, but don't rely on them to counteract bad eating habits.

Q Should I take supplements on the days I'm not training?
Yes. You get stronger as you recover from exercise, so making

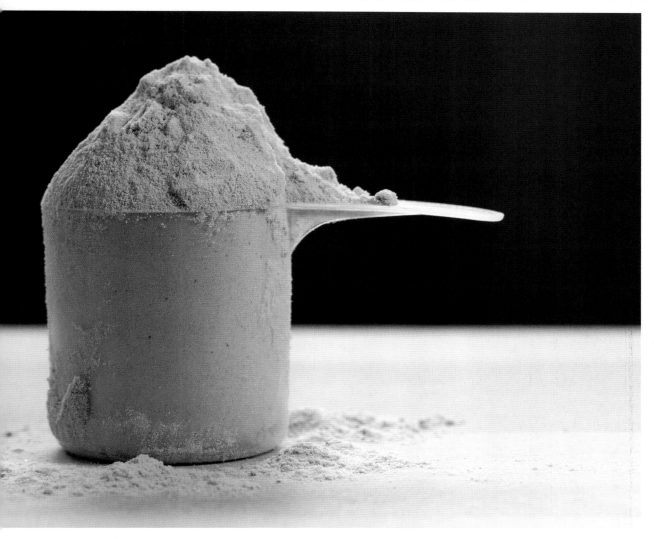

sure you're getting enough nutrients on rest days is essential.

Q Should I be waking in the middle of the night to take supplements?

Almost certainly not. You might have heard about bodybuilders getting up at 3am to neck a quick shake, but as soon as you're awake for more than three seconds you disrupt the production of melatonin, which is one of the most important hormones in getting to sleep. You're better off having some nice slow-digesting protein – such as raw nuts, cottage cheese or a casein shake – before bed.

Q Are supplements safe?

Since sports supplements are technically classified as food, they aren't subject to the same strict manufacturing, safety

testing or labelling as licensed medicines, so there's no guarantee they're living up to their claims. The EU is currently looking into the situation with a view to introducing stricter guidelines, but in the meantime it's up to individual manufacturers to maintain the quality of their own products. Look for supplements that are ISO17025 certified, which means they've been subjected to rigorous checks during their production.

Q Can I get ripped without working out if I take the right supplements?

Sadly, no. Anyone who tells you otherwise is fibbing. Eat right, train hard, tailor your supplement use to your goals and choose well-researched and tested products, and you'll see the results you want.

GET LEAN

Discover the best supplements for adding lean muscle mass

WHEY PROTEIN

WHAT The post-workout protein

WHY Whey is a fast-release protein, which means it's digested quickly and gets into your bloodstream – and your muscles – fast. What you consume after training is one of the most important meals you eat, so make sure you buy a high-quality whey protein.

HOW Your muscles are most receptive to nutrients as soon as you finish training, so drink a protein shake as soon as you've completed your final rep. Aim for a minimum of 30g of whey protein powder.

CASEIN

WHAT The bedtime protein

WHY Chances are you're already getting a fair hit of casein as it makes up around 80% of cow's milk. It's a slow-release protein, which means you get a 'drip-feed' effect over a longer period. This makes it unsuitable for taking straight after a workout when you need an instant hit of nutrients, but it's ideal for consuming just before you go to bed.

HOW Have it in a shake with either water or milk before turning in for the night. This will mean your muscles receive quality protein while you are sleeping, which is when your muscles are repaired and rebuilt.

BCAAS

WHAT The muscle pill

WHY Branched-chain amino acids, or BCAAs, are the best supplement to take during workouts because they help to keep a steady supply of proteins flowing into your muscles. This helps with muscle building as it reduces the amount of muscle loss during exercise and improves protein synthesis, the process by which new muscle tissue is built. BCAAs can also help to prevent muscle loss during periods of intermittent fasting.

HOW Take during your workouts.

CREATINE

WHAT The back-up generator

WHY Your body metabolises creatine into ATP, which is used for every initial muscle movement. It's therefore vital to have adequate supplies when you're doing heavy, high-intensity workouts in order to deliver the required energy to your muscles. In other words, creatine helps you lift harder for longer.

HOW Take 2-10g in your post-workout shake to replenish lost stores. Alternatively, split your dose and have half before your workout and half afterwards. And make sure you drink plenty of water with it: creatine is hygroscopic, which means it will suck water into your muscles and can leave you dehydrated.

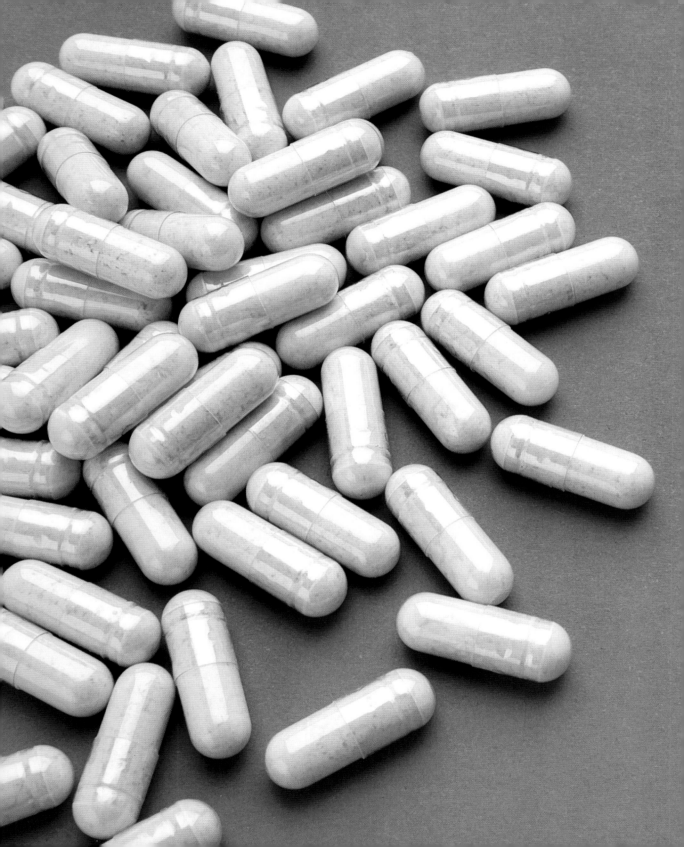

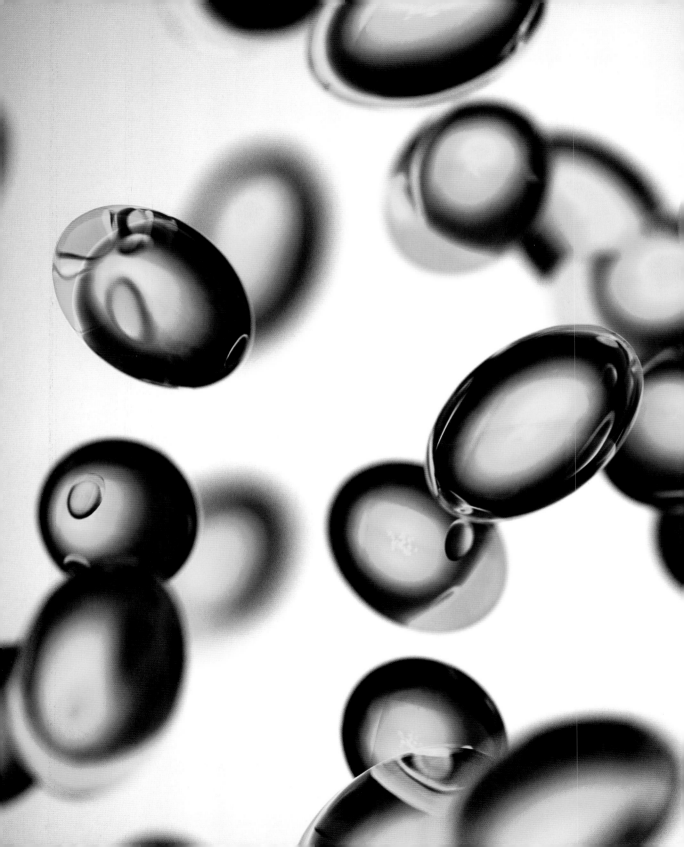

BEST OF THE REST

Use these supplements for better health and performance

FISH OIL

WHAT The wonder fluid

WHY It's important to include omega 3 fats in your diet for health reasons, and a supplement can help you to maintain a good ratio of omega 3 to omega 6 – most of us consume too much of the latter. Studies have shown fish oil supplementation results in decreased body fat and reduced inflammation. It has also been linked with increased serotonin levels, more focus in training and less stress.

HOW Take a spoonful with meals. Most authorities recommend 1–4g a day, depending on how much oily fish is already included in your diet.

MAGNESIUM

WHAT The body calmer

WHY Every organ needs magnesium, especially the heart, muscles and kidneys. If you skimp on this vital mineral you can experience anxiety, sleep problems and irritability. Magnesium also helps to maintain a normal heart rhythm and aids in the body's energy production.

HOW Stick to the recommended dose of less than 350mg a day and remember to take it with food – taking magnesium on an empty stomach can lead to diarrhoea and an upset stomach. Or you can use a magnesium spray or lotion.

ZINC

WHAT The masculine mineral

WHY Zinc is vital for your health and immune system. Our bodies aren't able to store it so you need to top up regularly.

HOW The RDA for zinc is 11mg for adult males – take no more than 40mg per day. Don't take it with coffee or foods containing phytates – such as wholegrains – because they can block its absorption. For the best benefits, take it with animal proteins as they promote absorption.

VITAMIN D

WHAT The sun substitute

WHY You should get your vitamin D from the sun, but that's a forlorn hope for the average deskbound worker – 20 minutes' exposure is enough in the summer, but according to the National Institute of Health it's impossible to get enough come the winter. Deficiency is common and linked to lower strength levels and increased body fat. It has also been associated with a number of diseases, including cancer, diabetes and depression.

HOW Supplements are available in tablet form or as an oral spray. Official government recommendations are low – aim for 3,000IU a day, which has been proved safe in multiple studies. It's fat-soluble, so take it with a meal.

PHASE 1

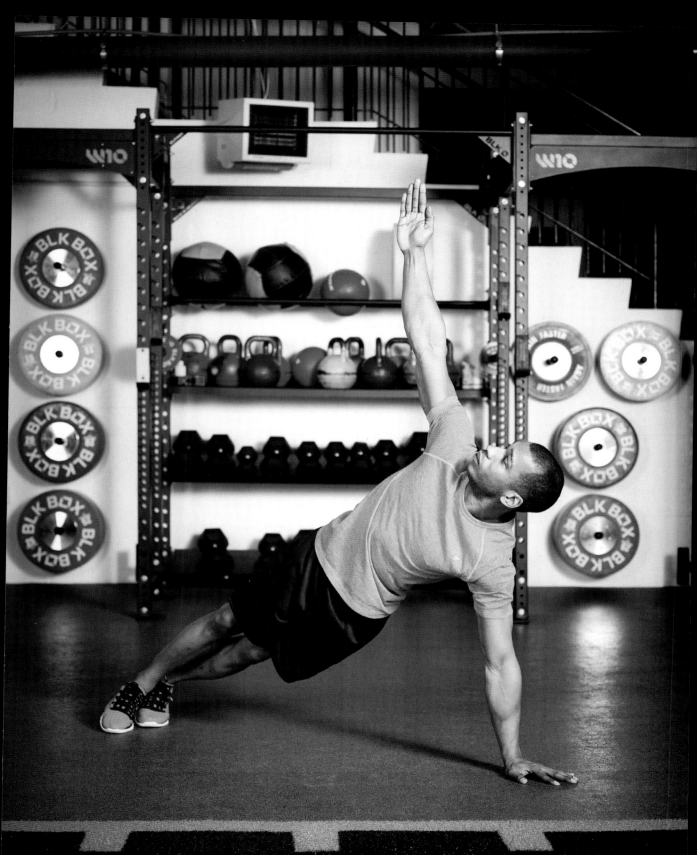

START STRONG

Here's the theory behind the first four weeks of the plan

The first phase of this eight-week plan lasts for four weeks and is composed of two two-week blocks. Each week involves three workouts and each of those workouts is a circuit, which means you do one set of each exercise in order before resting and then performing the sequence of moves again. The reason we're starting with circuits is because they're great for increasing your heart rate and maximising calorie burn, which will be key for losing fat. In the next phase you'll focus more on building lean muscle but, for now, all you need to do is follow the exercise instructions and give every workout everything you've got. Good luck!

PROGRAMME

Each circuit in first week of the plan is a whole-body session that includes a mixture of both bodyweight and dumbbell exercises. There are a couple of significant reasons for this. Whole-body workouts are an accessible way to train. As you progress you can concentrate more on specific muscle groups such as your chest and back but, when you're starting out, doing multiple moves that work the same muscle group can cause you to fatigue quickly and compromise the volume of work that you can complete in a workout. The circuits in the first week involve doing one upper body move followed by a lower body move. This will allow one muscle group to recover while the other is working while simultaneously posing a significant challenge to your heart and lungs.

PROGRESSION

The workouts in week two involve doing the same exercises in the same order as week one. That's not because we're lazy, it's because it will allow your body to take advantage of the neural adaptations (a flash way of describing your body's response to a physical challenge) so you can do more reps and lift more weight. You will perform two extra reps for each exercise and you'll have 30 seconds less rest at the end of each circuit. That may not seem like a lot but you should notice a difference. And if you're feeling really good you can increase the weight slightly. Your general aim should be to feel like you can just about complete the workout but if someone asked you to do more then you'd want to raise a little while flag.

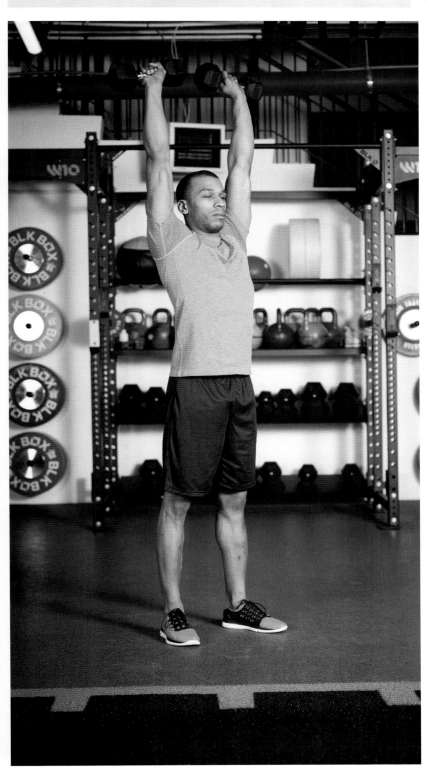

BLOCK TWO

The second fortnight of the plan is similar to the first two weeks in the sense that you do three circuit-style workouts per week. But this time each of the three workouts involves a different item of kit - either a kettlebell, medicine ball or barbell. One of the benefits of doing a circuit that involves just one item of kit is that you minimise the difficulty of changing between exercises so you can easily stick to your 10-second rest periods. Week four is the same as week three in terms of exercise selection and order but, again, it has been made more challenging to ensure that you are pushed outside of your comfort zone. As in week two, we've added two reps to each exercise and reduced the rest at the end of each circuit. You'll hate us at the time but thank us later.

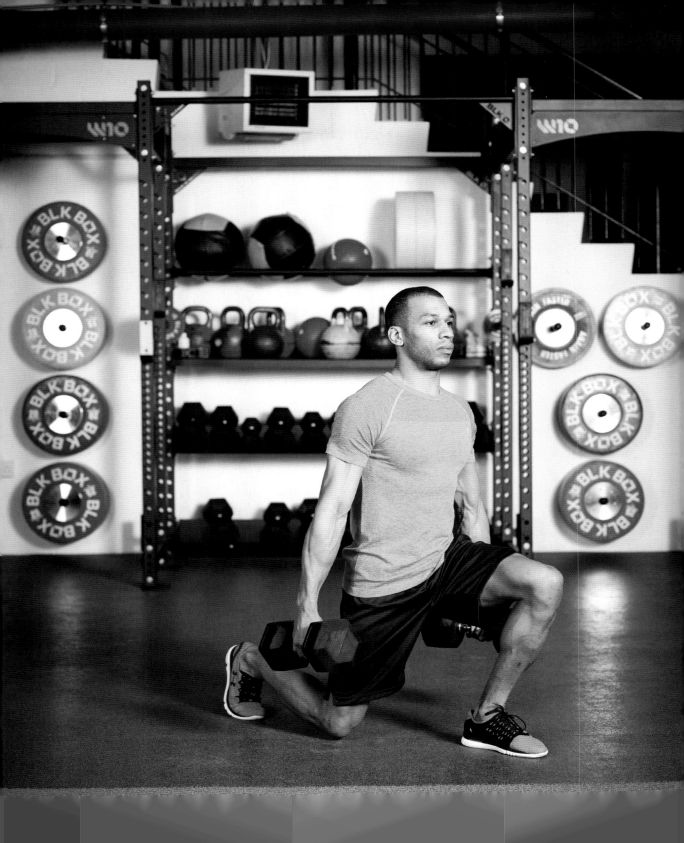

WEEK 1

MEAL PLAN

Monday

BREAKFAST
50g smoked salmon, ½ avocado, cherry tomatoes

SNACK
Post-workout shake: blend 1 scoop protein powder, 250ml milk, 1tsp almond butter, ½ banana and ice

LUNCH
100g quinoa mixed with chopped spring onion, crushed garlic, 1 chopped green chilli and pine nuts, served with cooked prawns

SNACK
Guacamole made with ¼ tomato, lime juice, ¼ red onion, coriander and ½ ripe avocado, served with sugar snap peas

DINNER
Chicken and cashew nut stir-fry with brown rice

SNACK
Greek yoghurt with cinnamon and a small handful of brazil nuts

Tuesday

BREAKFAST
Two scrambled eggs, spinach and a handful of mixed nuts

SNACK
50g cottage cheese with celery, carrot and cucumber sticks

LUNCH
Ham salad with ½ avocado

SNACK
100g beef jerky

DINNER
1 cod fillet, a small serving of new potatoes and a large serving of roasted vegetables

SNACK
Greek yoghurt with cinnamon and a small handful of almonds

Wednesday

BREAKFAST
Two scrambled eggs with smoked salmon, steamed kale and ½ avocado

SNACK
Post-workout shake: blend 1 scoop protein powder, 250ml milk, 1tsp almond butter, a handful of blueberries and ice

LUNCH
Smoked salmon with spinach, cucumber and mixed salad leaves

SNACK
Guacamole made with ¼ tomato, lime juice, ¼ red onion, coriander and ½ ripe avocado, served with red pepper slices

DINNER
1 salmon fillet with brown rice, green beans and asparagus

SNACK
Whey protein mixed with 1tbsp Greek yoghurt, water and ice

Thursday

BREAKFAST
Spinach and goat's cheese omelette with a handful of almonds

SNACK
Small pot of hummus with sugar snap peas, carrots and celery

LUNCH
Roast chicken with baked sweet potato and broccoli

SNACK
1 apple and 25g of peanut butter

DINNER
2 homemade hamburgers with a spinach and cherry tomato salad

SNACK
Greek yoghurt with cinnamon and a small handful of almonds

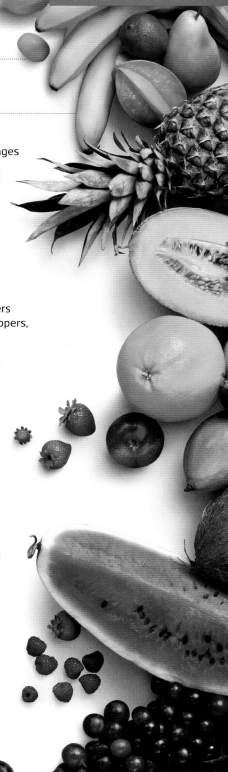

Friday

BREAKFAST
Two scrambled eggs
on brown toast

SNACK
Post-workout shake: blend
1 scoop protein powder,
230ml milk, 1tsp almond
butter, ½ banana and ice

LUNCH
Tuna and three-bean salad

SNACK
Guacamole made with
¼ tomato, lime juice, ¼
red onion, coriander and
½ ripe avocado, served
with sugar snap peas

DINNER
Grilled peppercorn
ribeye steak and Dijon
butter, served with
grilled mushrooms and
tomatoes and steamed
green vegetables

SNACK
Greek yoghurt with
cinnamon and a small
handful of macadamia nuts

Saturday

BREAKFAST
Bacon, 2 scrambled
eggs, grilled mushrooms
and tomatoes

SNACK
Small pot of hummus
with celery, courgette
and cucumber sticks

LUNCH
Baked sweet potato
with goat's cheese and
spring onions, served
with a side salad

SNACK
2 boiled eggs

DINNER
Chicken stir-fry
with beansprouts and
mixed vegetables

SNACK
Greek yoghurt with
cinnamon and a small
handful of almonds

Sunday

BREAKFAST
2 grilled chicken sausages
and 2 scrambled eggs,
small portion of baked
beans

SNACK
50g cottage cheese
with celery, carrot and
cucumber sticks

LUNCH
Lamb grilled on skewers
with green and red peppers,
cherry tomatoes and
red onion, served with
½ baked sweet potato

SNACK
1 can of tuna

DINNER
1 grilled salmon
fillet with roasted
vegetables

SNACK
Greek yoghurt with
cinnamon and a small
handful of macadamia
nuts

WORKOUT 1 FULL BODY CIRCUIT

DO 4 CIRCUITS IN TOTAL

1 Squat

REPS 10 **REST** 10sec

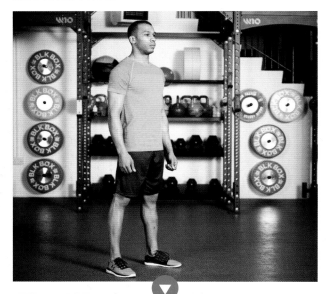

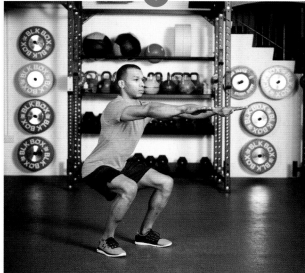

FORM Stand with your chest up and core braced. Bend your knees to squat down until your thighs are at least parallel to the ground, then press down through your heels to return to the start.

2 Overhead press

REPS 10 **REST** 10sec

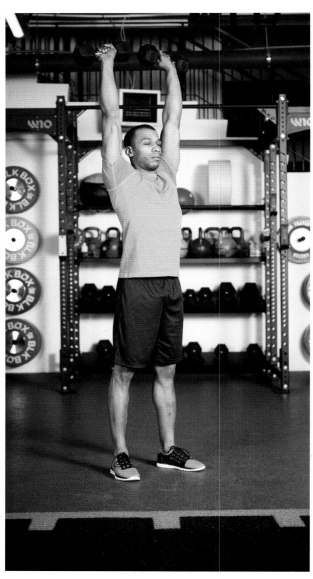

FORM Stand tall with your chest up and core braced, holding a dumbbell in each hand at shoulder height with palms facing forwards. Press the weights directly overhead so your arms are straight, then return slowly to the start.

3 Dumbbell lunge

REPS 10 REST 10sec

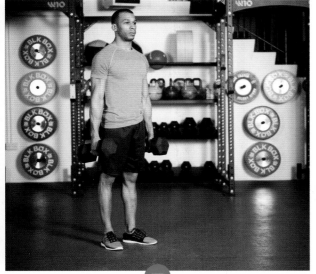

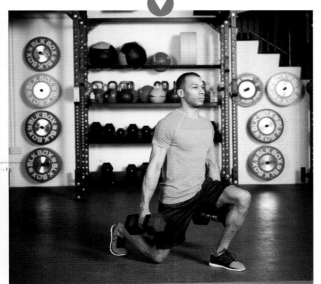

FORM Stand with chest up and core braced, holding a dumbbell in each hand. Take a step forward until both knees are at 90°. Push back off your front foot to return to the start. Repeat, leading with your other leg. Alternate sides.

4 Press-up

REPS 10 REST 10sec

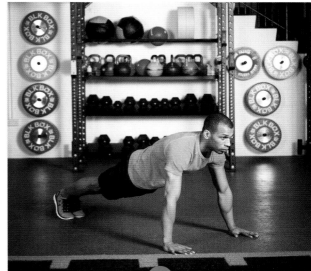

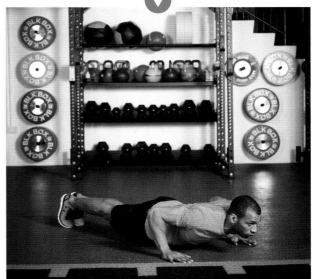

FORM Start in the press-up position with hands directly underneath your shoulders, your core and glutes braced, and feet together. Bend your elbows to lower your chest to the ground, then press back up powerfully to return to the start.

WORKOUT 1 FULL BODY CIRCUIT

5 Glute bridge

REPS 10 **REST** 10sec

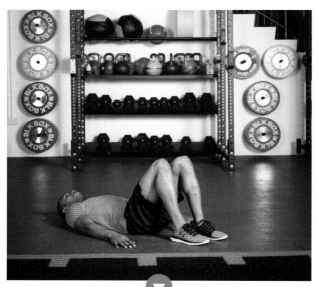

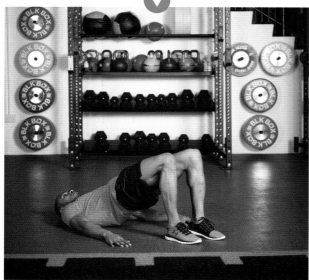

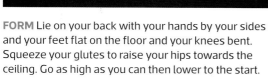

FORM Lie on your back with your hands by your sides and your feet flat on the floor and your knees bent. Squeeze your glutes to raise your hips towards the ceiling. Go as high as you can then lower to the start.

6 Bent over row

REPS 10 **REST** 2mins

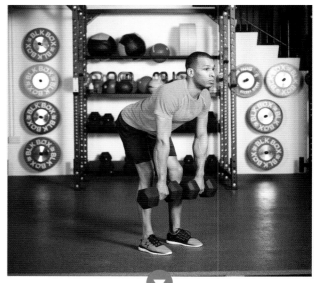

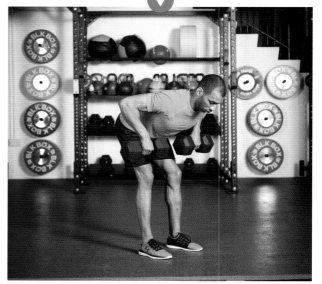

FORM Stand tall with your chest up and core braced, holding a dumbbell in each hand. Bend forwards – hingeing at the hips, not the waist – then row the weights up to your sides, leading with your elbows. Lower back to the start.

WORKOUT 1 ABS SUPERSET

Do 3 rounds of this superset after you have completed all four rounds of the main circuit

1A Straight-arm crunch

REPS 10 REST 10sec

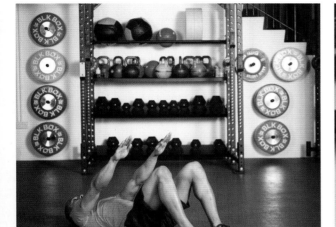

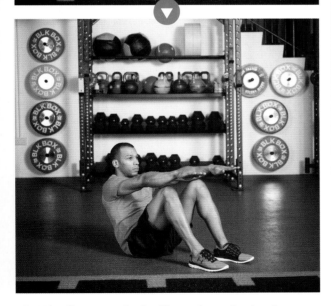

FORM Lie flat on your back with your knees bent and your arms straight. Crunch upward, pausing at the top of the movement, then lower back to the start.

1B Plank

TIME 30sec REST 60sec

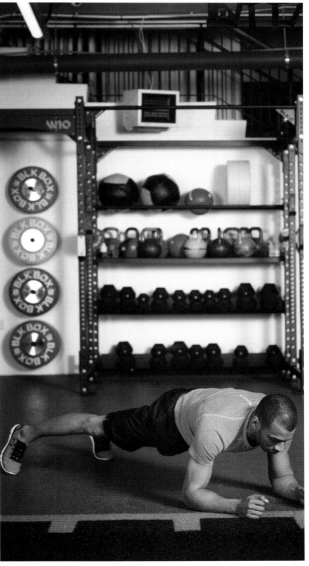

FORM Make sure your body is in a straight line from head to heels. Your elbows should be directly below your shoulders and your weight should be distributed evenly across your feet and forearms. Hold the position.

WORKOUT 2 FULL BODY CIRCUIT

DO 4 CIRCUITS IN TOTAL

1 Dumbbell squat

REPS 10 **REST** 10sec

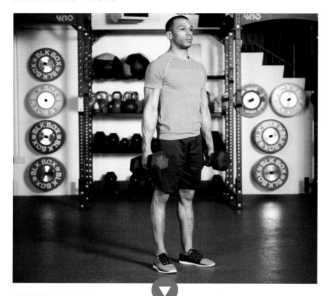

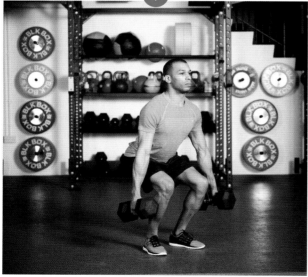

FORM Stand with your chest up and core braced, holding a dumbbell in each hand. Bend your knees to squat down until your thighs are at least parallel to the ground, then press down through your heels to return to the start.

2 Arnold press

REPS 10 **REST** 10sec

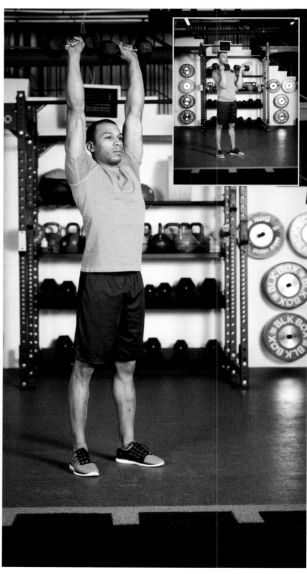

FORM Stand tall, holding a dumbbell in each hand by your shoulders with your palms facing you. Press the weights directly overhead. As you do so, rotate your wrists to finish with your palms facing forwards.

3 Reverse lunge

REPS 10 **REST** 10sec

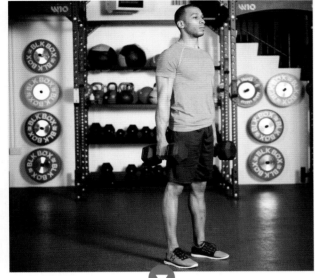

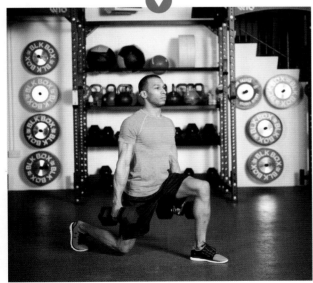

FORM Stand tall, holding a dumbbell in each hand. Take a big step backwards and bend your knees until they are both bent at 90°. Push back up to the start and repeat the move on the other side. Alternate sides.

4 Spiderman press-up

REPS 10 **REST** 10sec

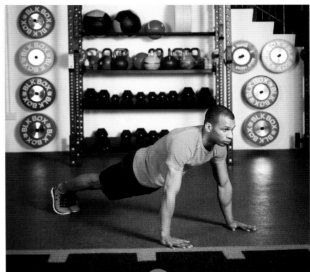

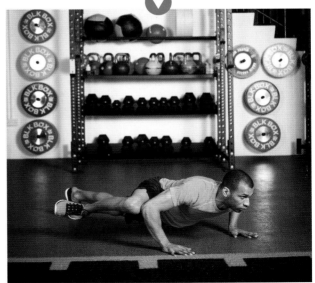

FORM Start at the top of a conventional press-up. As you lower towards the floor, bring one knee up towards your elbow. As you press back up, return to the start and alternate sides each rep.

WORKOUT 2 FULL BODY CIRCUIT

5 One-leg glute bridge

REPS 10 **REST** 10sec

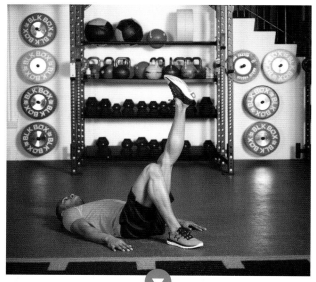

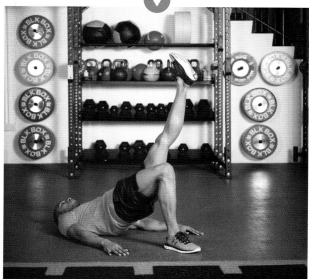

FORM Lie on your back with one foot on the floor with your knee bent and the other one straight and raised. Squeeze your glutes to raise your hips towards the ceiling. Lower to the start and alternate sides each rep.

6 Renegade row

REPS 10 **REST** 2mins

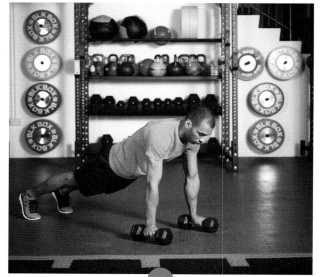

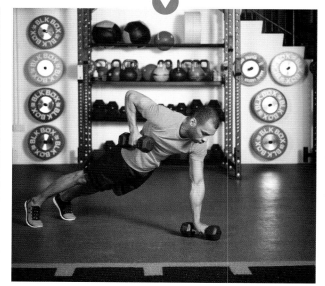

FORM Start in the top of the press-up position while holding a dumbbell in each hand. Contract your abs and raise one dumbbell up to your side, leading with your elbow. Lower and alternate sides each rep.

40

WORKOUT 2 ABS SUPERSET

Do 3 rounds of this superset after you have completed all four rounds of the main circuit

1A Reverse crunch

REPS 10 **REST** 10sec

1B Plank

TIME 30sec **REST** 60sec

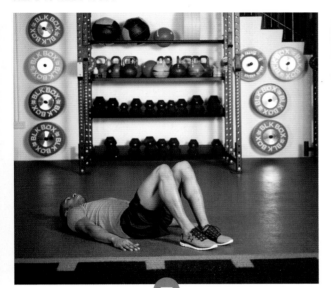

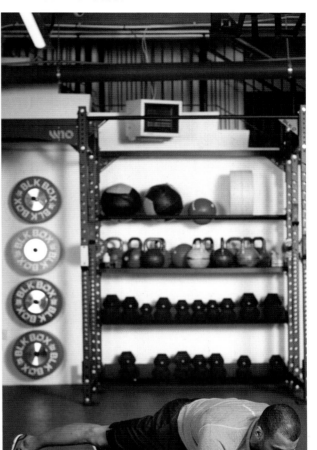

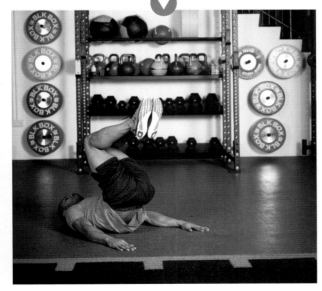

FORM Lie flat on your back with knees bent and arms flat against the floor. Contract your lower abs to draw your knees in towards your chest. Pause at the top of the move

FORM Make sure your body is in a straight line from head to heels. Your elbows should be directly below your shoulders and your weight should be distributed evenly across your feet and forearms. Hold the position.

WORKOUT 3 FULL BODY CIRCUIT

DO 4 CIRCUITS IN TOTAL

1 Squat jump

REPS 10 REST 10sec

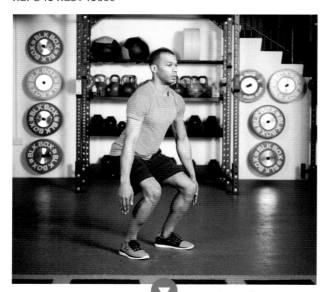

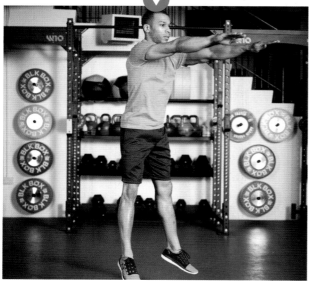

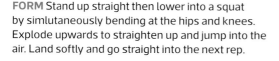

FORM Stand up straight then lower into a squat by simlutaneously bending at the hips and knees. Explode upwards to straighten up and jump into the air. Land softly and go straight into the next rep.

2 Lateral raise

REPS 10 REST 10sec

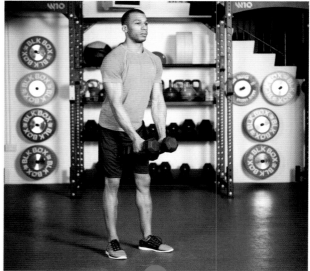

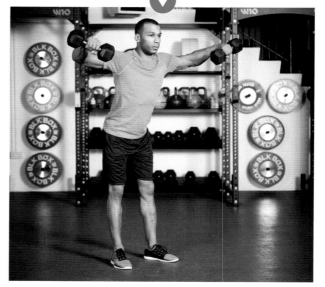

FORM Stand tall with your chest up and core braced, holding a dumbbell in each hand. Raise the weights out to the sides, leading with your elbows, until they reach shoulder height. Lower them slowly to return to the start.

3 Split squat

REPS 10 **REST** 10sec

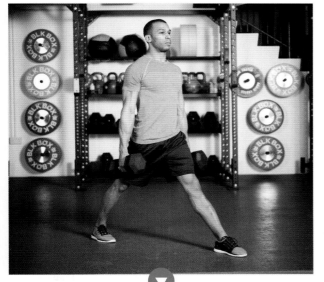

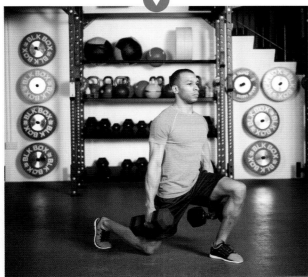

FORM Start with a dumbbell in each hand with your feet facing forwards a stride apart. Simultaneously bend both knees to lower towards the floor then press back up to the start. Swap sides each circuit.

4 T press-up

REPS 10 **REST** 10sec

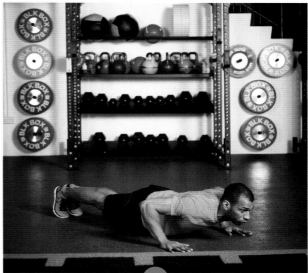

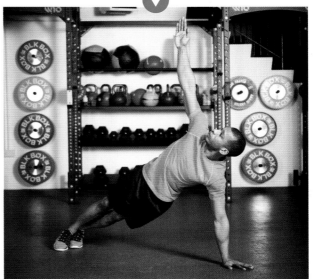

FORM Start in the top of a press-up position, lower your chest towards the floor, then press back up and rotate to open up your body and raise one arm up into the air. Return to the start and swap sides each rep.

WORKOUT 3 FULL BODY CIRCUIT

5 Romanian deadlift

REPS 10 **REST** 10sec

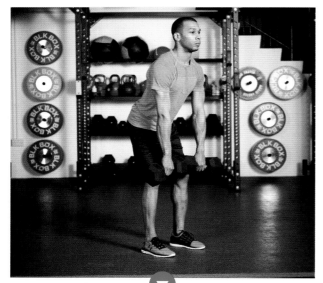

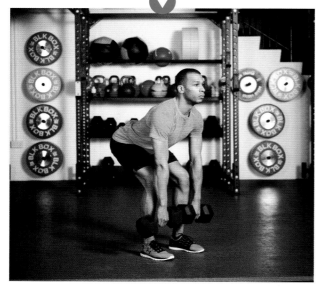

FORM Stand with a dumbbell in each hand resting on the front of your thighs. Hinge at the hips by pushing your bum backwards to send the weights down your thighs until you feel a strong hamstring stretch then stand back up.

6 Reverse grip bent-over row

REPS 10 **REST** 2mins

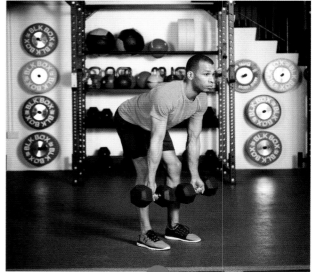

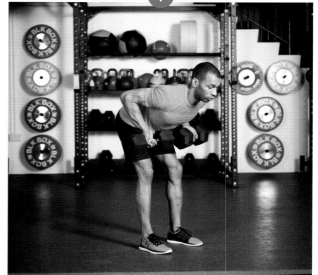

FORM Stand tall with your chest up and core braced, holding a dumbbell in each hand with palms facing up. Hinge at the hips, not the waist – then row the weights up to your sides, leading with your elbows. Lower back to the start and repeat.

WORKOUT 3 ABS SUPERSET

Do 3 rounds of this superset after you have completed all four rounds of the main circuit

1A Halo

REPS 10 **REST** 10sec

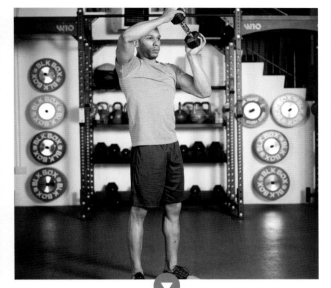

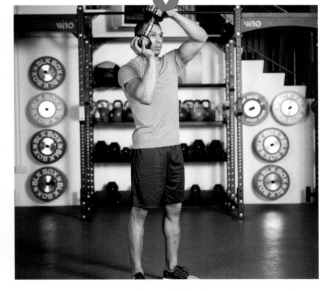

FORM Holding a dumbbell in both hands, move it around your head, engaging your core as you circle it around. After one complete circle, reverse directions.

1B Side plank

TIME 20sec (each side) **REST** 60sec

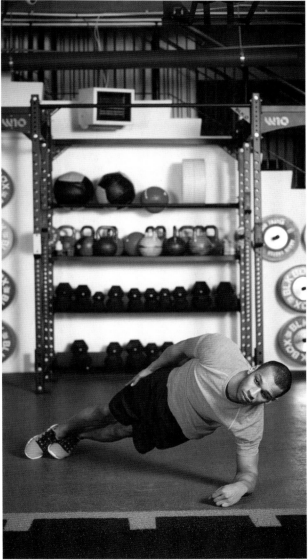

FORM Get onto one forearm with your feet "stacked" one on top of the other – or both on the floor, one behind the other (known as "staggered") if this is too hard. Keep your body in a straight line - once you start to sag, the set's over.

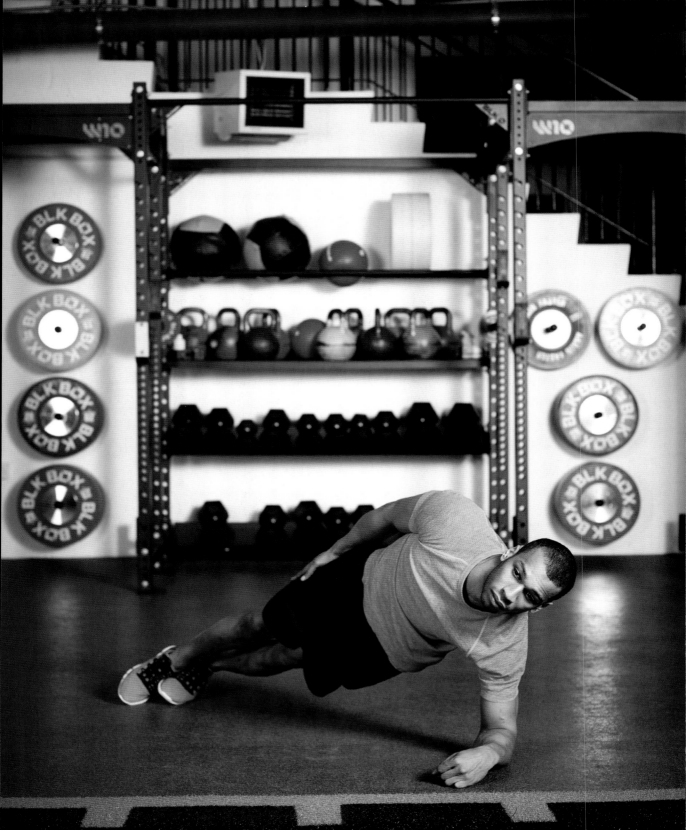

WEEK 2

MEAL PLAN

Monday

BREAKFAST
Roast chicken slices, spinach and a handful of mixed nuts

SNACK
Post-workout shake: blend 1 scoop protein powder, 200ml milk, 1tsp brazil nut butter and 1tbsp flax seeds

LUNCH
Grilled prawns with salad, avocado and pumpkin seeds

SNACK
2 boiled eggs

DINNER
Beef meatballs in tomato sauce, with, brown rice, spinach and green vegetables

SNACK
Greek yoghurt with cinnamon and a small handful of brazil nuts

Tuesday

BREAKFAST
2 boiled eggs, ½ avocado and asparagus

SNACK
Beef slices

LUNCH
Chicken and vegetable stir-fry with broccoli, onions and green peppers

SNACK
Guacamole and raw vegetables

DINNER
Chicken wrapped in Parma ham, with sweet potato mash and broccoli

SNACK
Greek yoghurt with cinnamon and a small handful of almonds

Wednesday

BREAKFAST
3-egg omelette with mixed peppers

SNACK
Post-workout shake: blend 1 scoop protein powder, 200ml milk, 1tsp brazil nut butter and 1tbsp flax seeds

LUNCH
2 homemade hamburgers (made with lean beef mince) with spinach salad, cherry tomatoes and chopped onion

SNACK
Guacamole and sliced red pepper

DINNER
Grilled turkey breast, with new potatoes, broccoli and mange tout

SNACK
Greek yoghurt with cinnamon and a small handful of brazil nuts

Thursday

BREAKFAST
Roast chicken slices, spinach and a handful of mixed nuts

SNACK
Ham and ½ avocado

LUNCH
Tuna salad, served with 1 baked sweet potato

SNACK
Greek yoghurt

DINNER
Steak with roasted vegetables

SNACK
50g cottage cheese with ½ punnet blueberries and 1tbsp pumpkin seeds

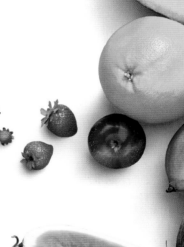

Friday

BREAKFAST
2 poached eggs, smoked salmon and ½ avocado

SNACK
Post-workout shake: blend 1 scoop protein powder, 200ml milk, 1tsp brazil nut butter and 1tbsp flax seeds

LUNCH
Grilled prawns with salad, avocado, quinoa and pumpkin seeds

SNACK
Guacamole and sliced red pepper

DINNER
Cod fillet with new potatoes, asparagus and green beans; 1 glass red wine

SNACK
Greek yoghurt with cinnamon and a small handful of brazil nuts

Saturday

BREAKFAST
2 scrambled eggs, ½ can reduced salt and sugar beans, tomatoes, mushrooms and 2 rashers grilled bacon

SNACK
1tbsp peanut butter and an apple

LUNCH
Chicken and vegetable stir-fry with broccoli, onions and green peppers

SNACK
1 can tuna

DINNER
2 homemade hamburgers with spinach salad, cherry tomatoes and chopped onion

SNACK
Whey protein mixed with 1tbsp Greek yoghurt, water and ice

Sunday

BREAKFAST
2 poached eggs, ½ an avocado mashed on 1 slice of toasted sourdough bread, tomatoes

SNACK
Smoked salmon and ½ avocado

LUNCH
Beef stir-fry

SNACK
1tbsp peanut butter and a banana

DINNER
Roast chicken, with new potatoes, broccoli, carrots, cabbage and gravy

SNACK
Whey protein mixed with 1tbsp Greek yoghurt, water and ice

WORKOUT 1 FULL BODY CIRCUIT

DO 4 CIRCUITS IN TOTAL

1 Squat

REPS 12 **REST** 10sec

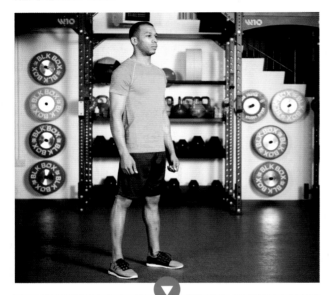

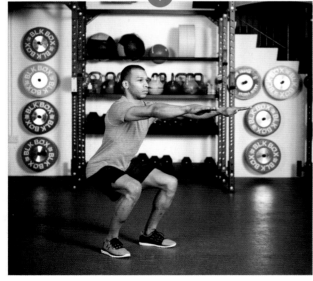

FORM Stand with your chest up and core braced. Bend your knees to squat down until your thighs are at least parallel to the ground, then press down through your heels to return to the start.

2 Overhead press

REPS 12 **REST** 10sec

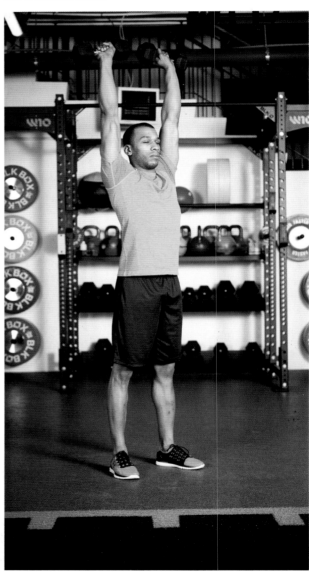

FORM Stand tall with your chest up and core braced, holding a dumbbell in each hand at shoulder height with palms facing forwards. Press the weights directly overhead so your arms are straight, then return slowly to the start.

3 Dumbbell lunge

REPS 12 **REST** 10sec

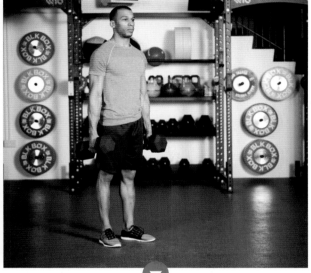

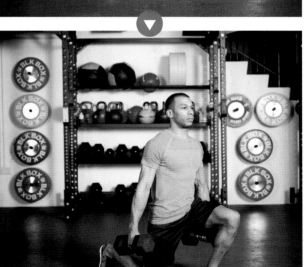

FORM Stand with chest up and core braced, holding a dumbbell in each hand. Take a step forward until both knees are at 90°. Push back off your front foot to return to the start. Repeat, leading with your other leg. Alternate sides.

4 Press-up

REPS 12 **REST** 10sec

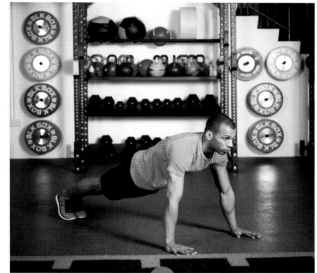

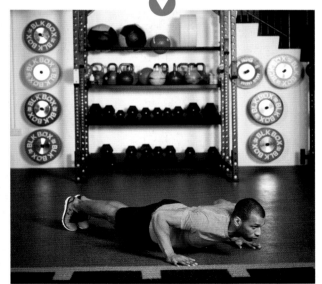

FORM Start in the press-up position with hands directly underneath your shoulders, your core and glutes braced, and feet together. Bend your elbows to lower your chest to the ground, then press back up powerfully to return to the start.

WORKOUT 1 FULL BODY CIRCUIT

5 Glute bridge

REPS 12 **REST** 10sec

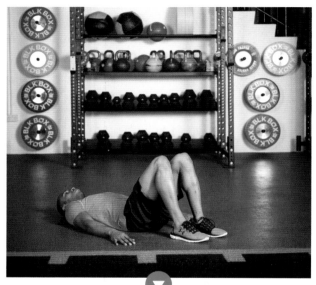

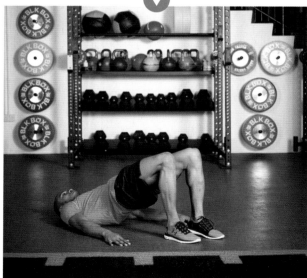

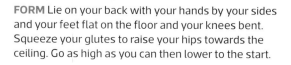

FORM Lie on your back with your hands by your sides
and your feet flat on the floor and your knees bent.
Squeeze your glutes to raise your hips towards the
ceiling. Go as high as you can then lower to the start.

6 Bent over row

REPS 12 **REST** 90secs

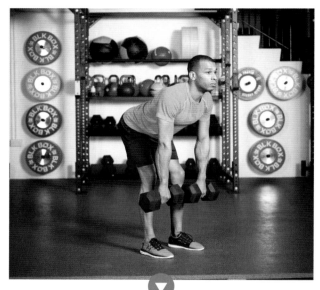

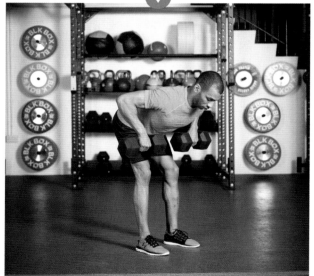

FORM Stand tall with your chest up and core braced, holding
a dumbbell in each hand. Bend forwards – hingeing at
the hips, not the waist – then row the weights up to your
sides, leading with your elbows. Lower back to the start.

WORKOUT 1 ABS SUPERSET

Do 3 rounds of this superset after you have completed all four rounds of the main circuit

1A Straight–arm crunch

REPS 12 **REST** 10sec

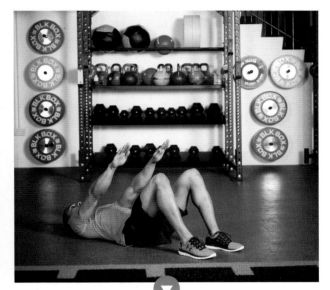

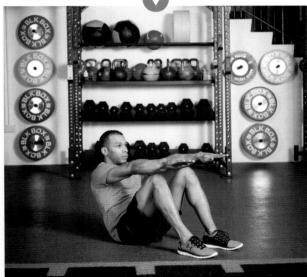

FORM Lie flat on your back with your knees bent and your arms straight. Crunch upward, pausing at the top of the movement, then lower back to the start.

1B Plank

TIME 40sec **REST** 60sec

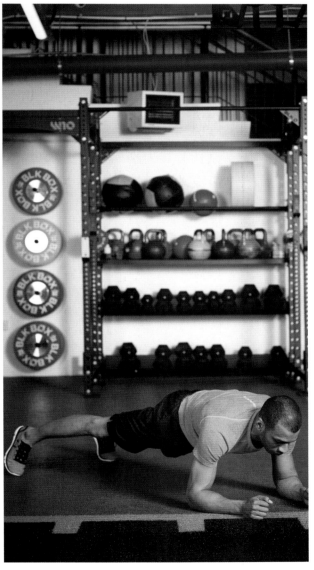

FORM Make sure your body is in a straight line from head to heels. Your elbows should be directly below your shoulders and your weight should be distributed evenly across your feet and forearms. Hold the position.

WORKOUT 2 FULL BODY CIRCUIT

DO 4
CIRCUITS
IN TOTAL

1 Dumbbell squat

REPS 12 **REST** 10sec

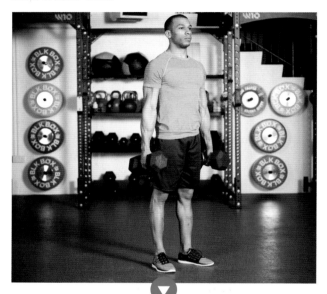

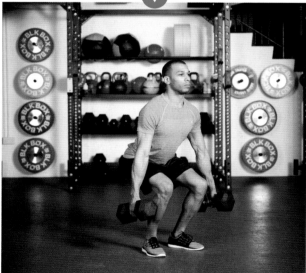

FORM Stand with your chest up and core braced, holding a dumbbell in each hand. Bend your knees to squat down until your thighs are at least parallel to the ground, then press down through your heels to return to the start.

2 Arnold press

REPS 12 **REST** 10sec

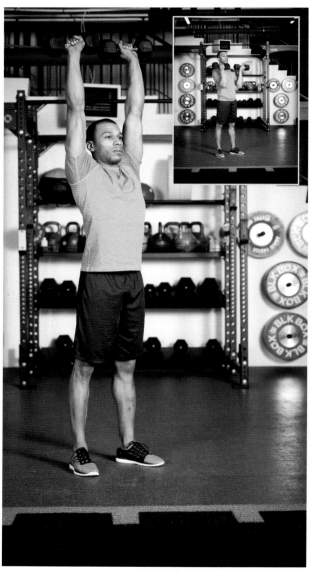

FORM Stand tall, holding a dumbbell in each hand by your shoulders with your palms facing you. Press the weights directly overhead. As you do so, rotate your wrists to finish with your palms facing forwards.

3 Reverse lunge

REPS 12 **REST** 10sec

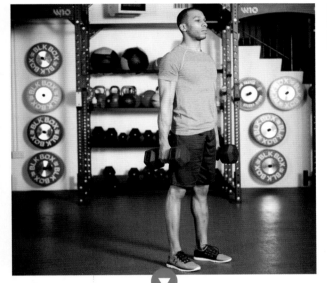

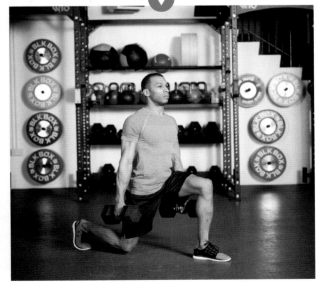

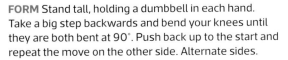

FORM Stand tall, holding a dumbbell in each hand. Take a big step backwards and bend your knees until they are both bent at 90°. Push back up to the start and repeat the move on the other side. Alternate sides.

4 Spiderman press-up

REPS 12 **REST** 10sec

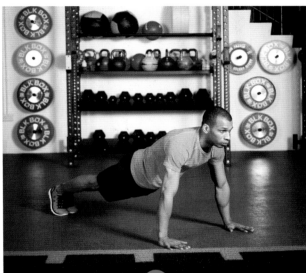

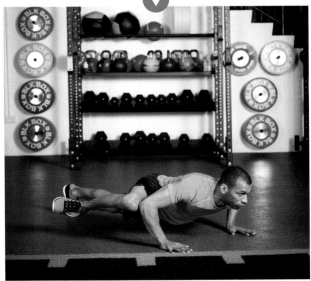

FORM Start at the top of a conventional press-up. As you lower towards the floor, bring one knee up towards your elbow. As you press back up, return to the start and alternate sides each rep.

WORKOUT 2 FULL BODY CIRCUIT

5 One-leg glute bridge

REPS 12 REST 10sec

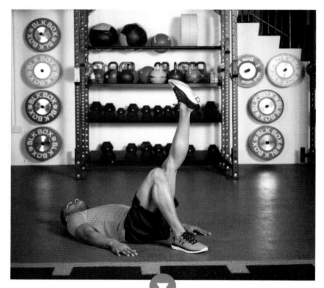

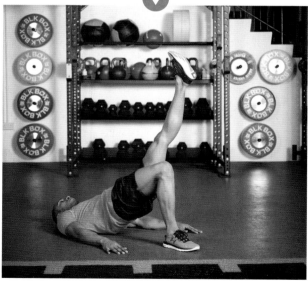

FORM Lie on your back with one foot on the floor with your knee bent and the other one straight and raised. Squeeze your glutes to raise your hips towards the ceiling. Lower to the start and alternate sides each rep.

6 Renegade row

REPS 12 REST 90secs

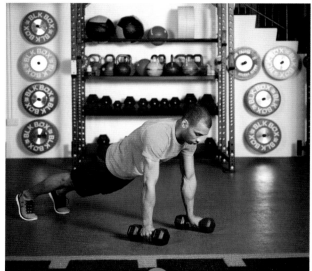

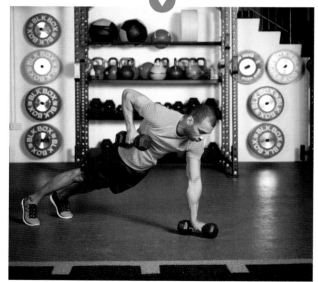

FORM Start in the top of the press-up position while holding a dumbbell in each hand. Contract your abs and raise one dumbbell up to your side, leading with your elbow. Lower and alternate sides each rep.

WORKOUT 2 ABS SUPERSET

Do 3 rounds of this superset after you have completed all four rounds of the main circuit

1A Reverse crunch

REPS 12 REST 10sec

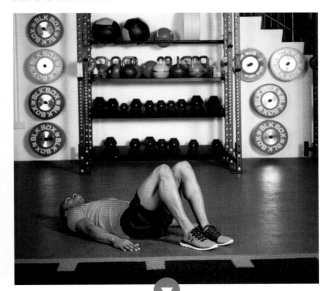

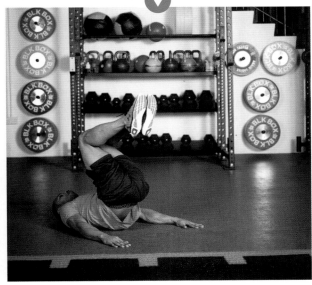

FORM Lie flat on your back with knees bent and arms flat against the floor. Contract your lower abs to draw your knees in towards your chest. Pause at the top of the move

1B Plank tap

TIME 40sec REST 60sec

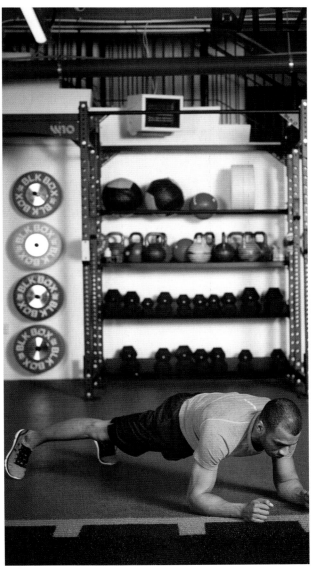

FORM Get into the plank position then raise one leg and place it approximately one foot away from the start position. Return to the start and perform the same movement on the other side.

WORKOUT 3 FULL BODY CIRCUIT

DO 4 CIRCUITS IN TOTAL

1 Squat jump

REPS 12 REST 10sec

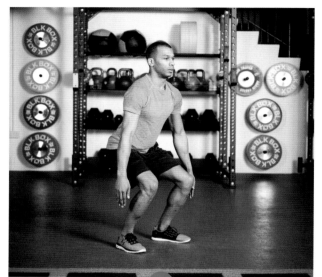

2 Lateral raise

REPS 12 REST 10sec

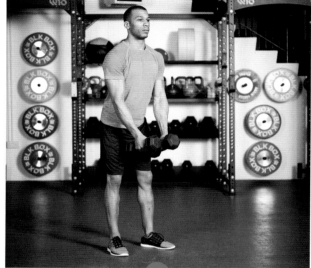

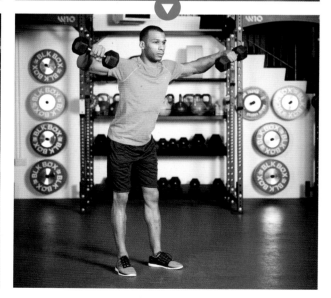

FORM Stand up straight then lower into a squat by simlutaneously bending at the hips and knees. Explode upwards to straighten up and jump into the air. Land softly and go straight into the next rep.

FORM Stand tall with your chest up and core braced, holding a dumbbell in each hand. Raise the weights out to the sides, leading with your elbows, until they reach shoulder height. Lower them slowly to return to the start.

3 Split squat

REPS 12 **REST** 10sec

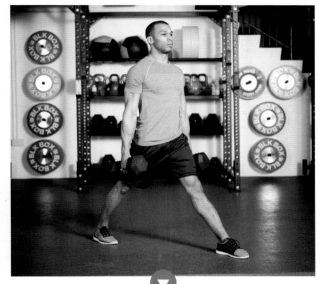

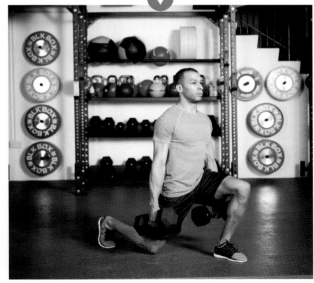

FORM Start with a dumbbell in each hand with your feet facing forwards a stride apart. Simultaneously bend both knees to lower towards the floor then press back up to the start. Swap sides each circuit.

4 T press-up

REPS 12 **REST** 10sec

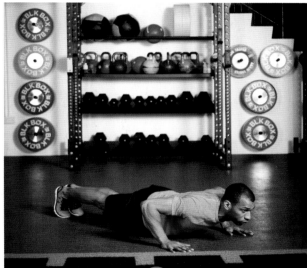

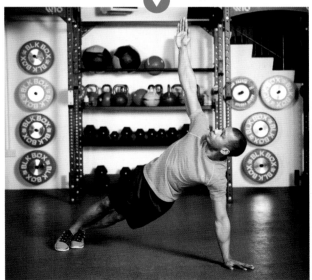

FORM Start in the top of a press-up position then rotate to open up your body and raise one arm up into the air until it is vertical then return to the start.

WORKOUT 3 FULL BODY CIRCUIT

5 Romanian deadlift

REPS 12 **REST** 10sec

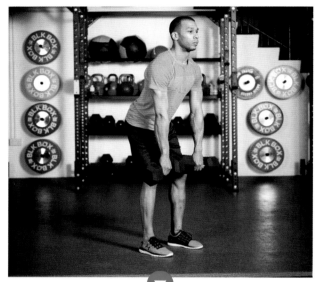

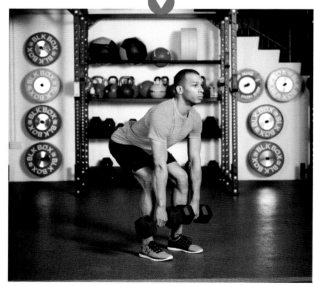

FORM Stand with a dumbbell in each hand resting on the front of your thighs. Hinge at the hips by pushing your bum backwards to send the weights down your thighs until you feel a strong hamstring stretch then stand back up.

6 Reverse grip bent–over row

REPS 12 **REST** 90sec

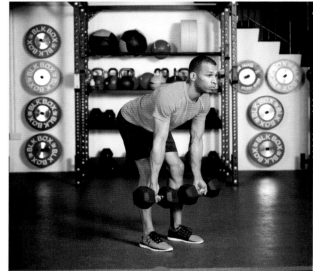

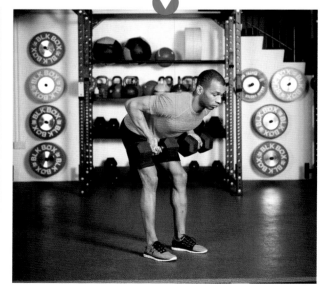

FORM Stand tall with your chest up and core braced, holding a dumbbell in each hand with palms facing up. Hinge at the hips, not the waist – then row the weights up to your sides, leading with your elbows. Lower back to the start and repeat.

WORKOUT 3 ABS SUPERSET

> Do 3 rounds of this superset after you have completed all four rounds of the main circuit

1A Halo

REPS 12 **REST** 10sec

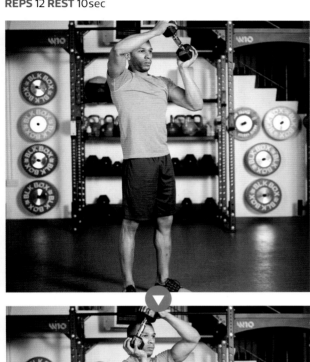

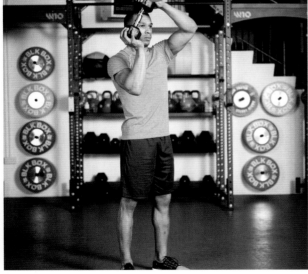

FORM Holding a dumbbell in both hands, move it around your head, engaging your core as you circle it around. After one complete circle, reverse directions.

1B Side plank

TIME 30sec (each side) **REST** 60sec

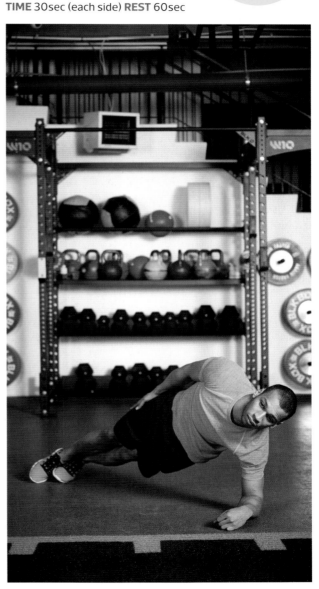

FORM Get onto one forearm with your feet "stacked" one on top of the other – or both on the floor, one behind the other (known as "staggered") if this is too hard. Keep your body in a straight line - once you start to sag, the set's over.

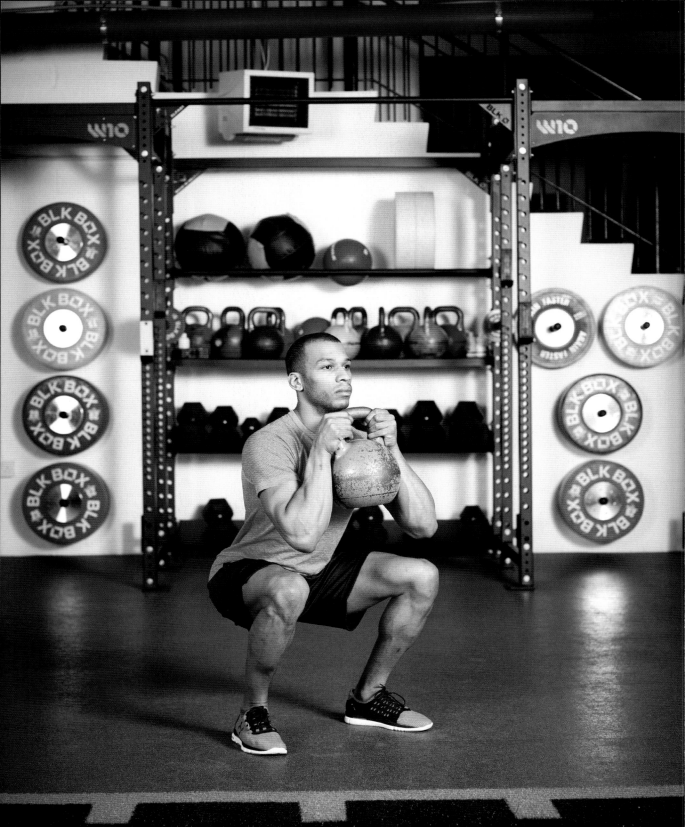

WEEK 3

MEAL PLAN

Monday

BREAKFAST
Roast chicken slices
with a bowl of grapes
and melon cubes

SNACK
Post-workout shake: blend 1
scoop protein powder, 100ml
milk, $\frac{1}{2}$ banana, 75ml semi-
skimmed milk and 1tbsp oats

LUNCH
1 medium sweet potato
with 1 can tuna in water
(drained) and spinach

SNACK
Small pot of hummus
with celery, carrot and
cucumber sticks

DINNER
Ginger chicken stir-fry

SNACK
Greek yoghurt with
cinnamon and a small
handful of pecan nuts

Tuesday

BREAKFAST
Two scrambled eggs, spinach
and a handful of mixed nuts

SNACK
Celery sticks, brazil nut
butter and 10 raisins

LUNCH
Grilled prawns with a wild
rice mixed salad, $\frac{1}{2}$ avocado
and pumpkin seeds

SNACK
100g beef jerky

DINNER
Chilli beef stuffed
peppers and side salad

SNACK
Greek yoghurt with
cinnamon and a small
handful of walnuts

Wednesday

BREAKFAST
2 poached eggs, smoked
salmon, steamed kale
and $\frac{1}{2}$ avocado

SNACK
Post-workout shake: blend
1 scoop protein powder, $\frac{1}{2}$
banana, raspberries, 150ml
skimmed milk, 100ml natural
yoghurt, 1tbsp sunflower
seeds and 20g rolled oats

LUNCH
Lamb steak with new
potatoes, a side salad
and cherry tomatoes

SNACK
Small pot of hummus
with celery, carrot and
cucumber sticks

DINNER
1 cod fillet with sweet potato
and steamed vegetables

SNACK
Greek yoghurt with
cinnamon and a small
handful of pecan nuts

Thursday

BREAKFAST
Spinach and goat's
cheese omelette and
a handful of almonds

SNACK
Celery sticks and
brazil nut butter

LUNCH
Grilled prawns, mixed
salad, $\frac{1}{2}$ avocado and
pumpkin seeds

SNACK
2 scrambled eggs
and spinach

DINNER
Tuna steak, new potatoes,
asparagus, broccoli
and cauliflower

SNACK
Greek yoghurt with
cinnamon and a small
handful of walnuts

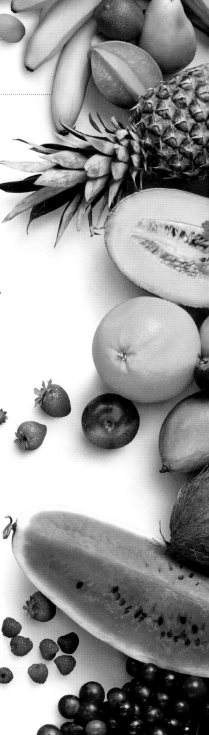

Friday

BREAKFAST
150g porridge oats cooked with 200ml semi-skimmed milk, ½ banana and 1tsp honey; stir in ½ scoop whey protein at the end

SNACK
Post-workout shake: blend 1 scoop protein powder, 100ml milk, ½ banana, 75ml semi-skimmed milk and 1tbsp oats

LUNCH
Ham and avocado salad

SNACK
Small pot of hummus with celery, carrot and cucumber sticks

DINNER
2 pork chops with sweet potato mash and green beans; 1 glass red wine

SNACK
Greek yoghurt with cinnamon and a small handful of pecan nuts

Saturday

BREAKFAST
2 scrambled eggs, 2 grilled sausages, grilled mushrooms and tomatoes

SNACK
Celery sticks with almond butter

LUNCH
100g quinoa mixed with 2 boiled eggs, 1 chicken breast and broccoli

SNACK
1 can of tuna

DINNER
Homemade beef chilli with green vegetables and cauliflower rice (sauté a chopped onion for 10 minutes, then blend in a food processor with small florets of 1 cauliflower for 5-6 minutes)

SNACK
Greek yoghurt with cinnamon and a small handful of walnuts

Sunday

BREAKFAST
2 poached eggs and smoked salmon

SNACK
A handful of brazil nuts

LUNCH
Diced lamb grilled on skewers with diced green and red peppers, diced onion and cherry tomatoes, with 1 baked sweet potato

SNACK
Ham and ½ avocado

DINNER
Grilled chicken breast with beetroot, spinach and goat's cheese salad

SNACK
Greek yoghurt with cinnamon and a small handful of walnuts

WORKOUT 1 KETTLEBELL CIRCUIT

DO 4 CIRCUITS IN TOTAL

1 Clean

REPS 10 REST 10sec

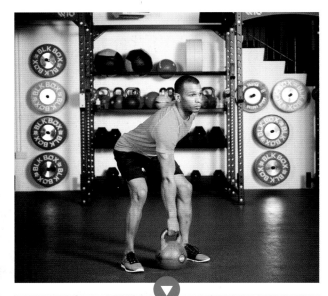

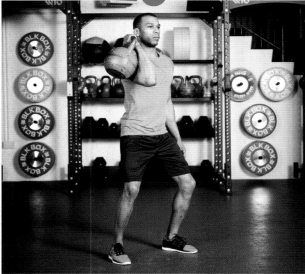

FORM Swing the kettlebell between your legs and drive the hips forwards. Once the bell passes stomach height, draw your elbow back and slide your hand under and around the bell to catch it in the "rack" position.

2 Overhead press

REPS 10 REST 10sec

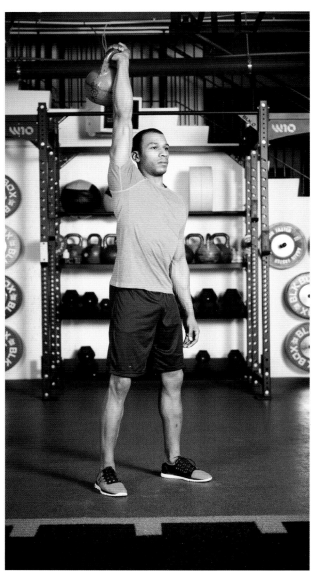

FORM Start in the rack position with the kettlebell at shoulder height and your elbow tucked in to your side. Press the weight overhead, using the most efficient path possible to reduce stress on your shoulder joint. Swap sides each circuit.

3 Windmill

REPS 10 **REST** 10sec

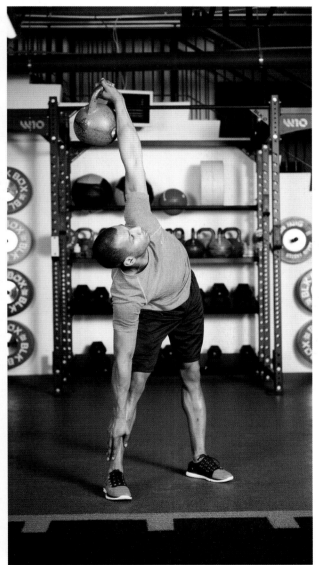

4 Goblet squat

REPS 10 **REST** 10sec

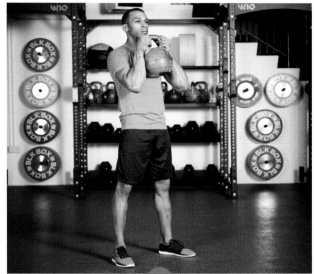

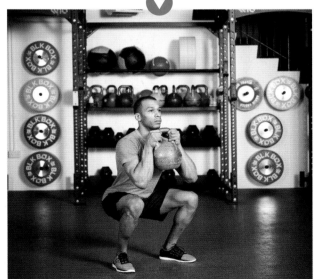

FORM Start with the weight above your head and your feet wider than shoulder-width apart with your weight distribution biased towards the side holding the bell. Keeping your eyes on the bell, lower your torso until your hand touches the floor.

FORM Hold your kettlebell in both hands, and squat down with your back straight and chest up. Descend until your elbows touch the insides of your knees, then put your weight on your heels as you stand back up.

WORKOUT 1 KETTLEBELL CIRCUIT

5 Around the world

REPS 10 REST 10sec

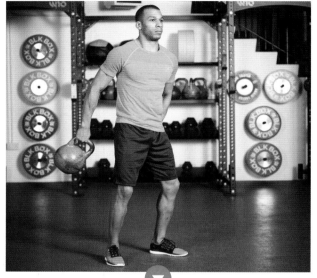

6 Plank drag

REPS 10 REST 2mins

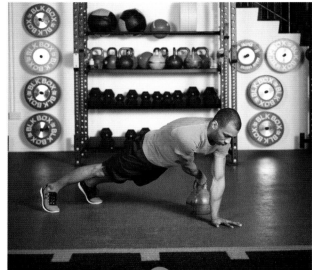

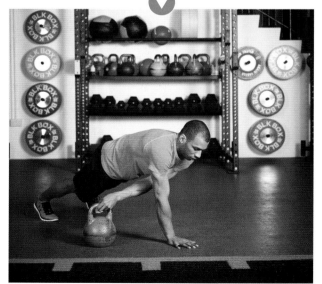

FORM Swing the kettlebell out and around your body, swapping hands in front of you and continuing to swing it around your body. Swap hands behind your back and continue that pattern. Change direction each circuit.

FORM Get into a straight-arm plank position with your body in a straight line from head to heels and position a kettlebell to one side of your body. Reach through with the opposite hand to drag the bell across to the other side.

WORKOUT 1 FINISHER

Swing super-century

THE CHALLENGE 100 swings as quickly as possible

Do 1 round of this finisher after you have completed all four rounds of the main circuit

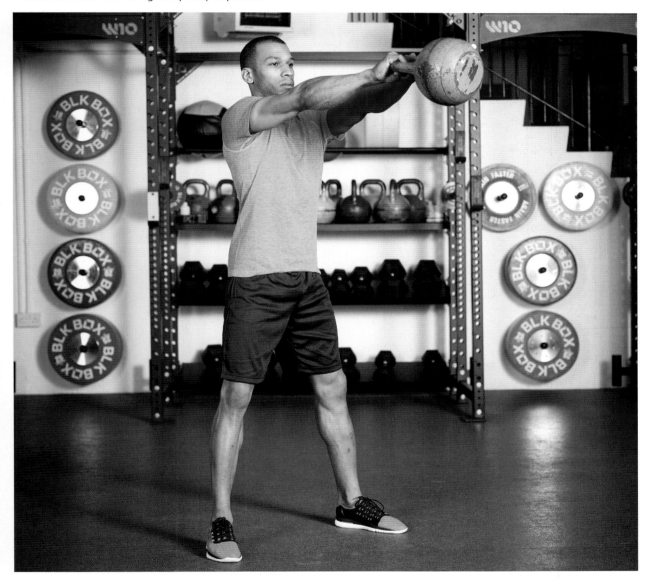

WHY **The kettlebell swing is the classic kettlebell exercise. This high-rep challenge will test your grip, strength, cardiovascular endurance and mental strength because you'll want to give up halfway through.**

HOW Swing the bell back between your legs then push your hips through explosively to swing the bell up to shoulder height. You can put the bell down when you need to rest but try to do it in as few sets as possible.

WORKOUT 2 MEDICINE BALL CIRCUIT

DO 4 CIRCUITS IN TOTAL

1 Squat

REPS 10 **REST** 10sec

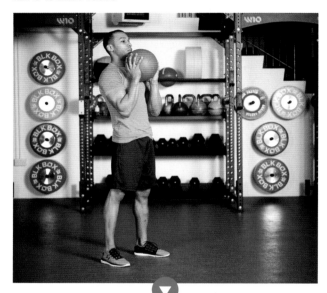

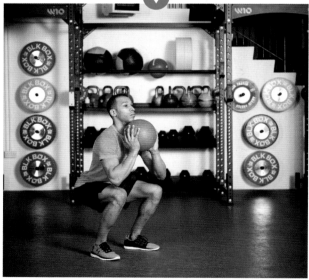

FORM Hold the ball in both hands. Keeping your chest up and core tight, squat down as low as you can. Push through your heels to stand back up.

2 Slam

REPS 10 **REST** 10sec

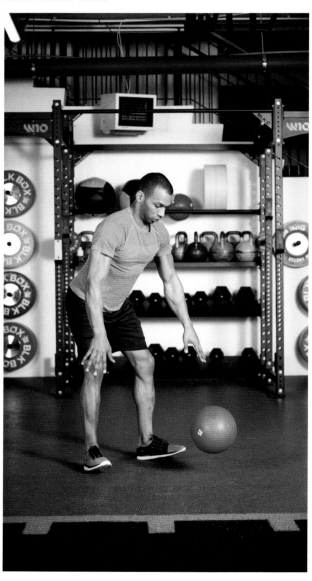

FORM Stand tall, holding the ball above your head. Slam it down powerfully to the floor in front of you, then pick it up and repeat.

3 Passing press-up

REPS 10 **REST** 10sec

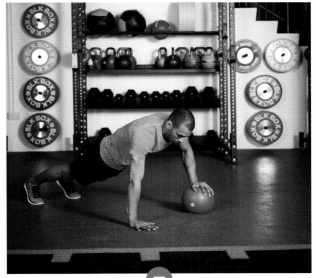

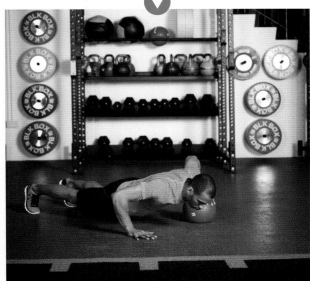

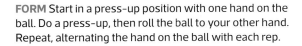

FORM Start in a press-up position with one hand on the ball. Do a press-up, then roll the ball to your other hand. Repeat, alternating the hand on the ball with each rep.

4 Lunge press

REPS 10 **REST** 10sec

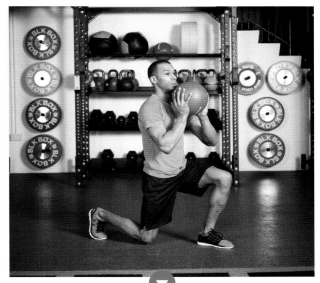

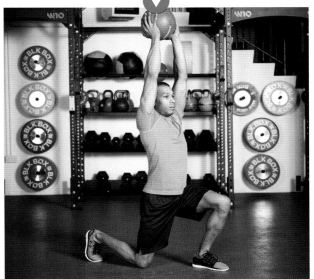

FORM Hold the ball in both hands then perform a lunge, pressing the ball directly overhead as you go. Lower it as you stand back up. Continue, alternating leading legs.

WORKOUT 2 MEDICINE BALL CIRCUIT

5 Leg raise

REPS 10 **REST** 10sec

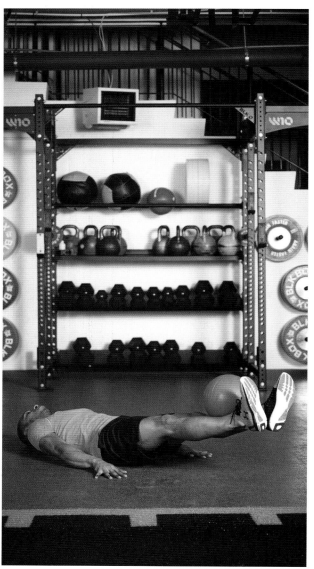

6 Standing Russian twist

REPS 10 **REST** 2mins

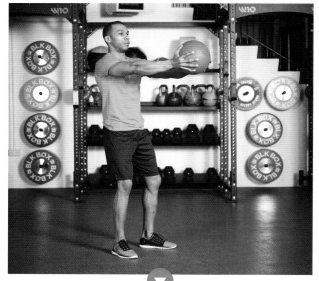

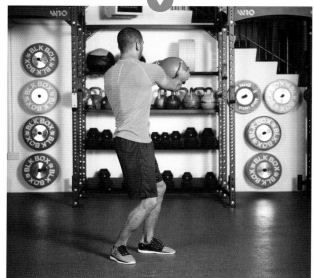

FORM Lie on your back with the ball between your ankles. Raise your legs up until they are vertical then lower them under control to the start position and repeat the exercise.

FORM Stand tall, holding the ball in both hands. Rotate to one side and then the other, keeping your abs engaged. That's one rep.

WORKOUT 2 FINISHER

Do 1 round of this finisher after you have completed all four rounds of the main circuit

Wall ball blast

CHALLENGE 50 wall throws as quickly as possible

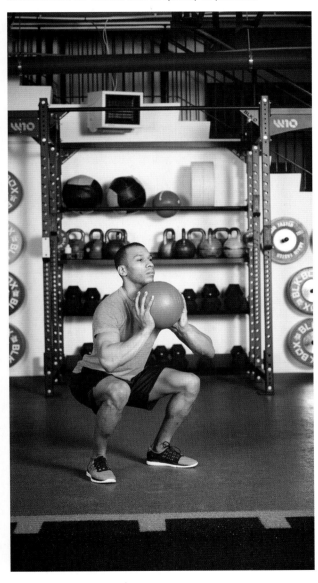

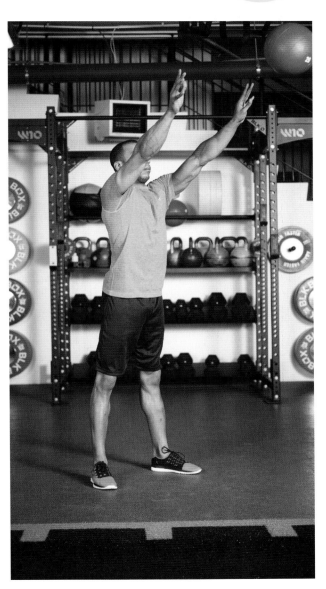

WHY This is a great test of your power endurance because you should aim to put maximum effort into each throw but, because the reps are high, you'll soon be suffering with the lactic acid build-up.

HOW Stand about one meter from a wall, go into a half squat then straighten up and throw the ball at the wall. Catch it and repeat the move, aiming to hit the same spot on the wall each time as a test of your coordination.

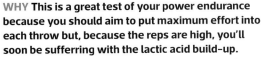

WORKOUT 3 BARBELL CIRCUIT

DO 4 CIRCUITS IN TOTAL

1 Deadlift

REPS 10 **REST** 10sec

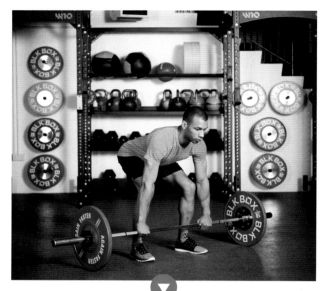

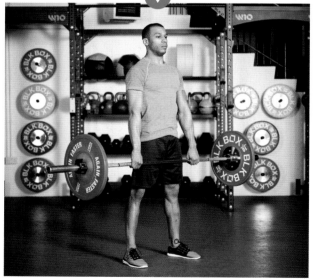

FORM Grasp the bar with your hands just outside your legs. Lift the bar by driving your hips forward, keeping a flat back. Lower the bar under control – though once you get up to really heavy weights, it's OK to drop the bar on your final rep.

2 Bent-over row

REPS 10 **REST** 10sec

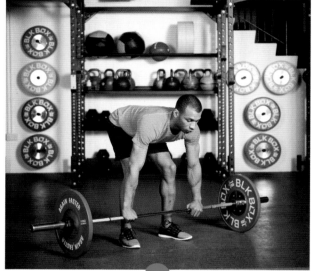

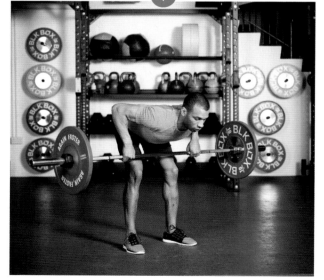

FORM Bend at the hips until you're at a roughly 45° angle to the floor. Pull the bar up to touch your belly button and then lower under control. If you're moving your upper body to shift the bar, the weight's too heavy.

3 Romanian deadlift

REPS 10 **REST** 10sec

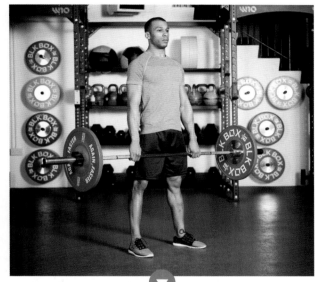

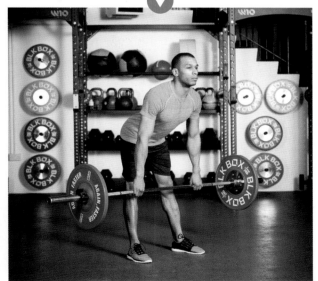

FORM Hold the bar with an overhand grip and push your backside back to send the bar down the front of your thighs. Lower until you feel a strong stretch in your hamstrings then straighten up to the start.

4 Clean

REPS 10 **REST** 10sec

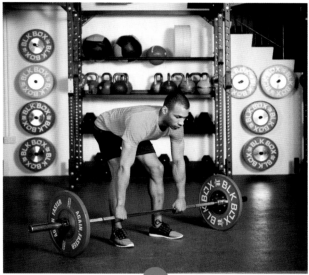

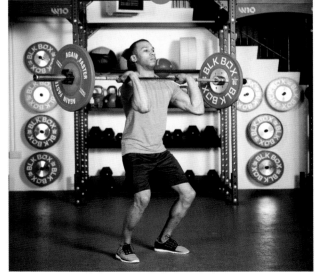

FORM Start by holding the bar with a shoulder-width grip in front of your thighs. Squat down slightly, then drive through your heels to explode upwards, using the momentum to help pull the bar up to chest height and catching it on your chest.

WORKOUT 3 BARBELL CIRCUIT

5 Front squat

REPS 10 **REST** 10sec

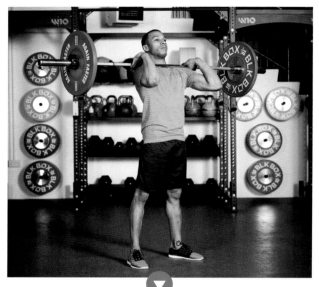

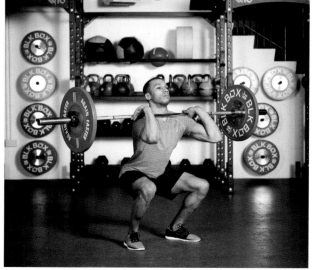

FORM Hold the bar on the front of your shoulders with your elbows high. Simultaneously bend at the hips and the knees, keeping your knees in line with your toes, to lower towards the floor then press back up to the start.

6 Overhead press

REPS 10 **REST** 2mins

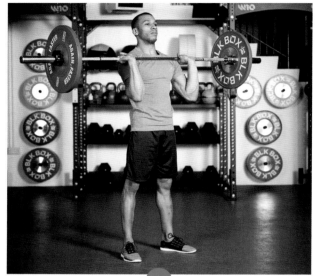

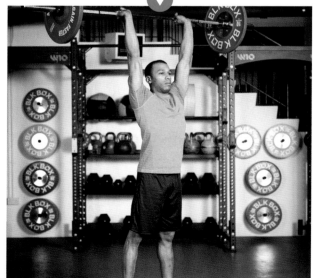

FORM With your feet shoulder-width apart, position a bar on your upper chest, gripping it with hands just wider than shoulder-width apart. Brace your abs as you press the bar straight upwards. Pause at the top, then lower.

WORKOUT 3 FINISHER

Do 1 round of this finisher after you have completed all four rounds of the main circuit

Squat death

CHALLENGE 50 squats as quickly as possible

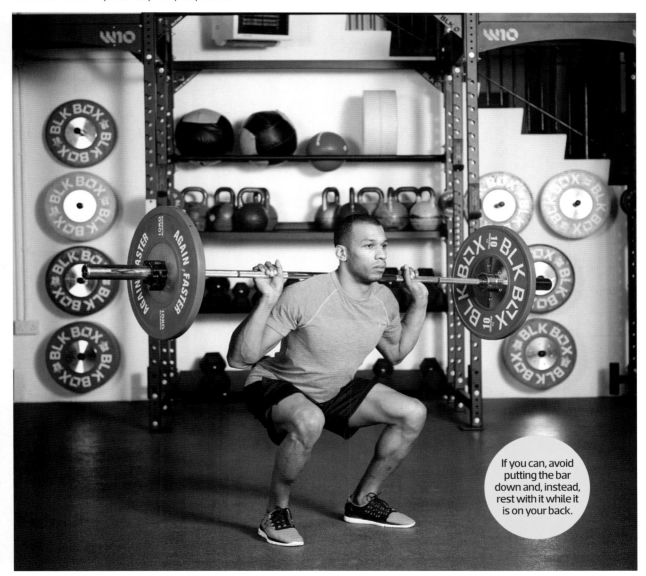

If you can, avoid putting the bar down and, instead, rest with it while it is on your back.

WHY You'll already be tired when you start this challenge so you'll quickly experience the burning sensation that signals a build up of lactic acid. It may not feel like cause for celebration but this is also great for burning fat.

HOW Perform a squat by simultaneously bending at the knees and hips to lower towards the floor, keeping your chest up and your weight on your heels and mid-foot. Aim to complete the reps in as few sets as possible.

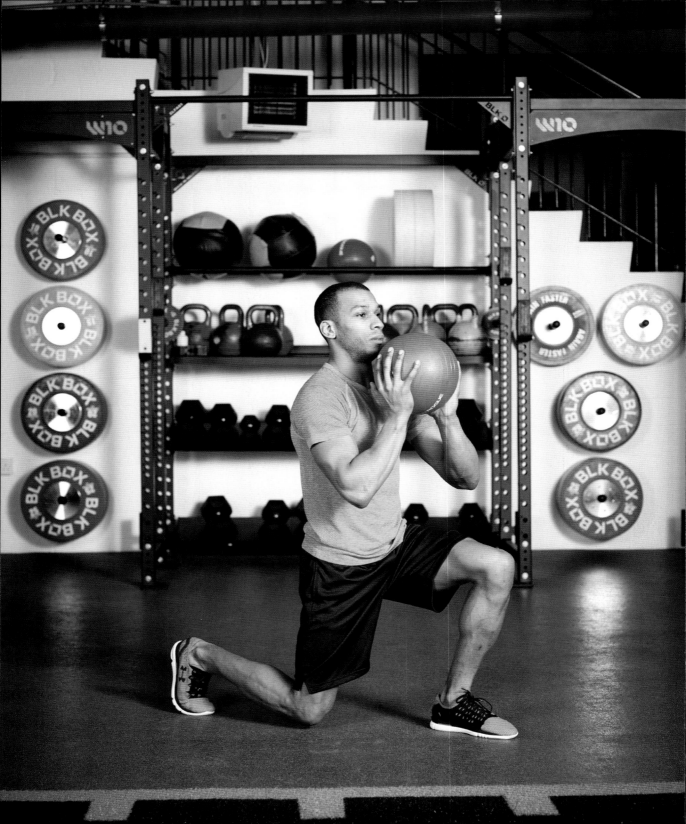

WEEK 4

MEAL PLAN

Monday

BREAKFAST
Spinach and goat's cheese omelette with a handful of almonds

SNACK
Post-workout shake: blend 150ml milk, 1 scoop chocolate whey protein powder, ½ banana and 2tbsp Greek yoghurt

LUNCH
Salmon fillet, 150g couscous and 150g Greek salad with sundried tomatoes, cucumber, red onion, feta cheese, olives, and 1 pepper

SNACK
Hummus, 1 carrot, 100g sliced green and red pepper

DINNER
Grilled chicken breast with chilli sauce and roasted vegetables

SNACK
100g cottage cheese and 2 wholegrain rice cakes

Tuesday

BREAKFAST
Roast beef slices with wilted spinach and asparagus

SNACK
Pineapple slices and cottage cheese

LUNCH
Grilled chicken breast with mixed salad and ½ avocado

SNACK
1 banana and a handful of almonds

DINNER
120g tuna steak, stir-fried broccoli, green beans and spinach

SNACK
Greek yoghurt and blueberries

Wednesday

BREAKFAST
2 boiled eggs and 1 slice rye bread

SNACK
Post-workout shake: blend 150ml milk, 1 scoop chocolate whey protein powder, ½ banana and 2tbsp Greek yoghurt

LUNCH
200g can tuna mixed with 2tsp chickpeas, lettuce, cucumber, spring onion, carrot, coriander, 30g (dry weight) cooked brown rice, olive oil and balsamic vinegar

SNACK
Apple and a handful of pumpkin seeds

DINNER
120g salmon, new potatoes, stir-fried broccoli, green beans, red pepper and spinach

SNACK
100g cottage cheese and 2 wholegrain rice cakes

Thursday

BREAKFAST
2 grilled sausages and 2 scrambled eggs

SNACK
Pineapple slices and cottage cheese

LUNCH
½ carton carrot and coriander soup with steamed green vegetables

SNACK
1 banana and a handful of almonds

DINNER
Large chicken salad with toasted walnuts

SNACK
Greek yoghurt with cinnamon and 6 brazil nuts

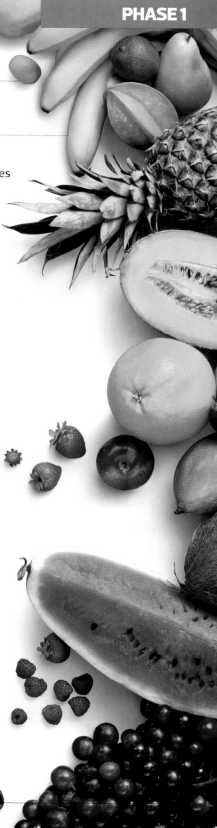

Friday

BREAKFAST
Roast chicken slices
and a handful of nuts

SNACK
Post-workout shake:
blend 150ml milk,
1 scoop chocolate whey
protein powder, ½ banana
and 2tbsp Greek yoghurt

LUNCH
Ham and avocado salad

SNACK
A handful of almonds, raisins
and dark chocolate chips

DINNER
Beef fajitas: 100g fillet
steak cut into strips with
1 red, 1 green pepper
and 2 tortilla wraps

SNACK
100g cottage cheese and
2 wholegrain rice cakes

Saturday

BREAKFAST
2 scrambled eggs, ½
can reduced salt and
sugar beans, tomatoes,
mushrooms and 2
rashers grilled bacon

SNACK
Pineapple slices and
cottage cheese

LUNCH
Tuna salad with cherry
tomatoes and beetroot

SNACK
1 banana and a handful
of almonds

DINNER
200g salmon teriyaki with
brown rice, spinach and
steamed courgette slices

SNACK
Greek yoghurt with
cinnamon and brazil nuts

Sunday

BREAKFAST
2 grilled chicken sausages
and 2 scrambled eggs,
small portion of baked
beans

SNACK
A handful of almonds
and raisins

LUNCH
½ carton of carrot
and coriander soup
with steamed
green vegetables

SNACK
Hummus with carrot
sticks and 100g sliced
green and red peppers

DINNER
Roast beef, sweet
potato mash,
carrots, spinach,
broccoli and parsnips

SNACK
115g cottage cheese
on 2 wholegrain
rice cakes

WORKOUT 1 KETTLEBELL CIRCUIT

DO 4 CIRCUITS IN TOTAL

1 Clean

REPS 12 **REST** 10sec

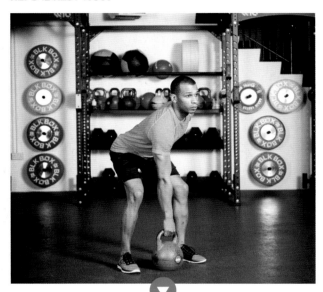

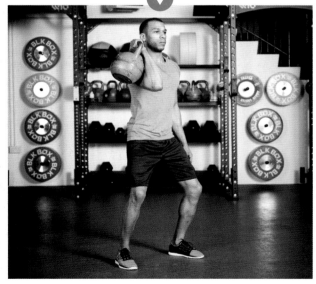

FORM Swing the kettlebell between your legs and drive the hips forwards. Once the bell passes stomach height, draw your elbow back and slide your hand under and around the bell to catch it in the "rack" position.

2 Overhead press

REPS 12 **REST** 10sec

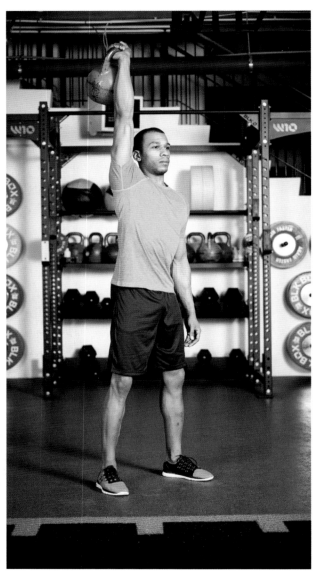

FORM Start in the rack position with the kettlebell at shoulder height and your elbow tucked in to your side. Press the weight overhead, using the most efficient path possible to reduce stress on your shoulder joint. Swap sides each circuit.

3 Windmill

REPS 12 **REST** 10sec

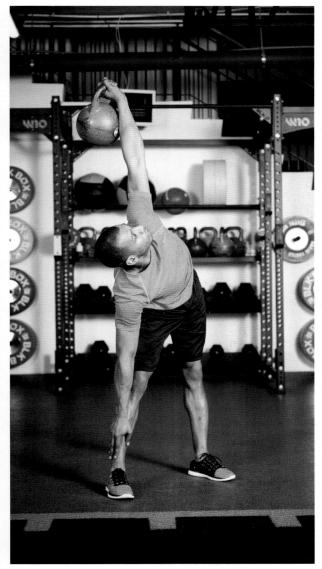

4 Goblet squat

REPS 12 **REST** 10sec

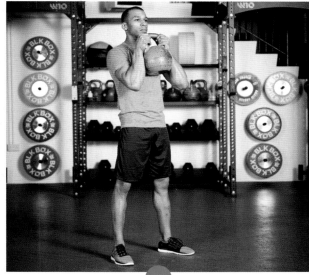

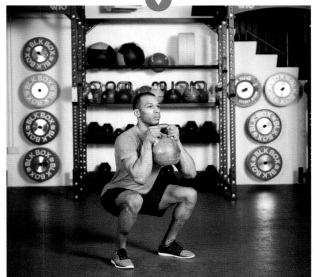

FORM Start with the weight above your head and your feet wider than shoulder-width apart with your weight distribution biased towards the side holding the bell. Keeping your eyes on the bell, lower your torso until your hand touches the floor.

FORM Hold your kettlebell in both hands, and squat down with your back straight and chest up. Descend until your elbows touch the insides of your knees, then put your weight on your heels as you stand back up.

WORKOUT 1 KETTLEBELL CIRCUIT

5 Around the world

REPS 12 **REST** 10sec

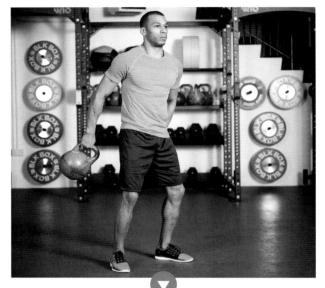

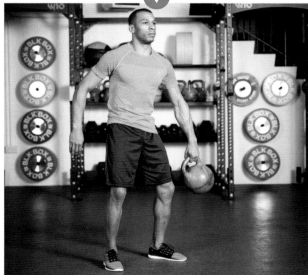

6 Plank drag

REPS 12 **REST** 90sec

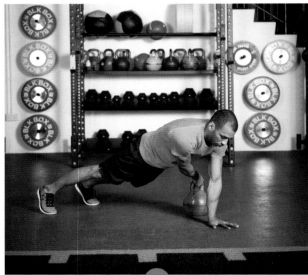

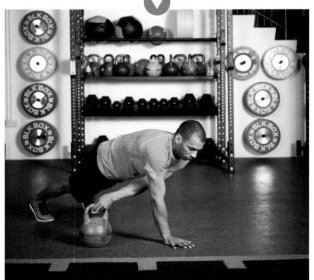

FORM Swing the kettlebell out and around your body, swapping hands in front of you and continuing to swing it around your body. Swap hands behind your back and continue that pattern. Change direction each circuit.

FORM Get into a straight-arm plank position with your body in a straight line from head to heels and position a kettlebell to one side of your body. Reach through with the opposite hand to drag the bell across to the other side.

WORKOUT 1 FINISHER

Do 1 round of this finisher after you have completed all four rounds of the main circuit

Swing super-century

THE CHALLENGE 100 swings as quickly as possible

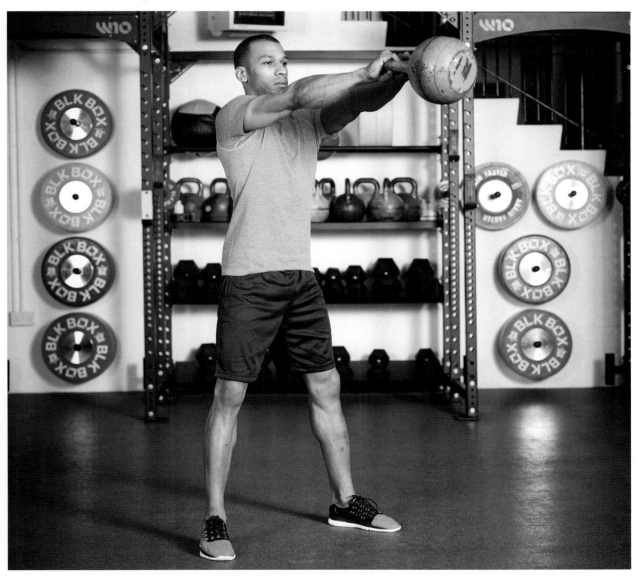

WHY The kettlebell swing is the classic kettlebell exercise. This high-rep challenge will test your grip, strength, cardiovascular endurance and mental strength because you'll want to give up halfway through.

HOW Swing the bell back between your legs then push your hips through explosively to swing the bell up to shoulder height. You can put the bell down when you need to rest but try to do it in as few sets as possible.

WORKOUT 2 MEDICINE BALL CIRCUIT

DO 4 CIRCUITS IN TOTAL

1 Squat

REPS 12 **REST** 10sec

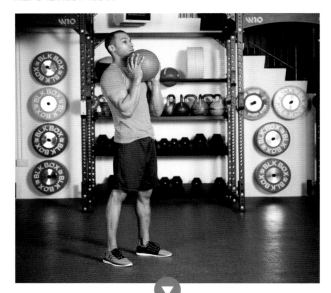

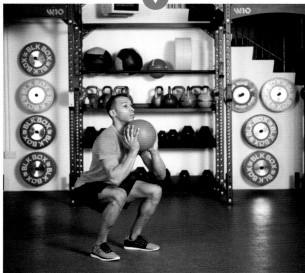

FORM Hold the ball in both hands. Keeping your chest up and core tight, squat down as low as you can. Push through your heels to stand back up.

2 Slam

REPS 12 **REST** 10sec

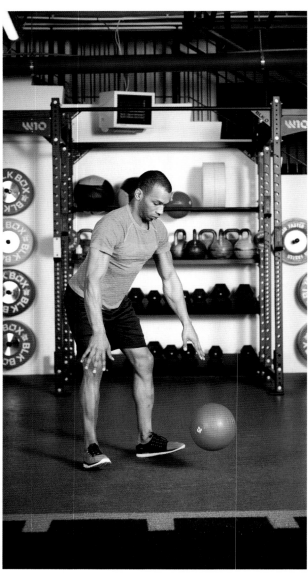

FORM Stand tall, holding the ball above your head. Slam it down powerfully to the floor in front of you, then pick it up and repeat.

3 Passing press-up

REPS 12 **REST** 10sec

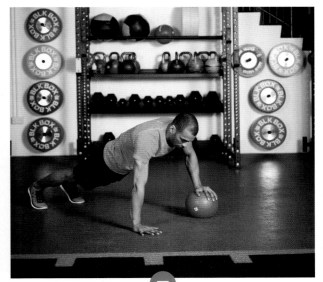

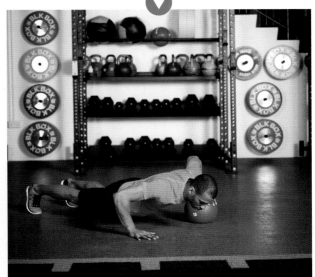

FORM Start in a press-up position with one hand on the ball. Do a press-up, then roll the ball to your other hand. Repeat, alternating the hand on the ball with each rep.

4 Lunge press

REPS 12 **REST** 10sec

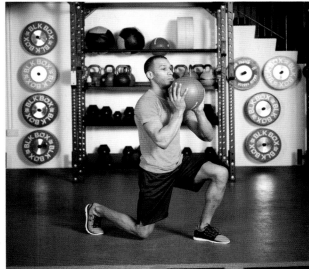

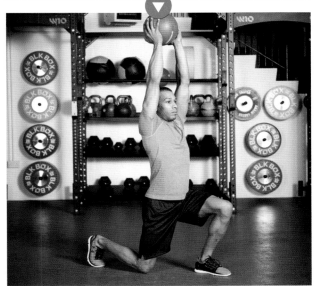

FORM Hold the ball in both hands then perform a lunge, pressing the ball directly overhead as you go. Lower it as you stand back up. Continue, alternating leading legs.

WORKOUT 2 MEDICINE BALL CIRCUIT

5 Leg raise

REPS 12 **REST** 10sec

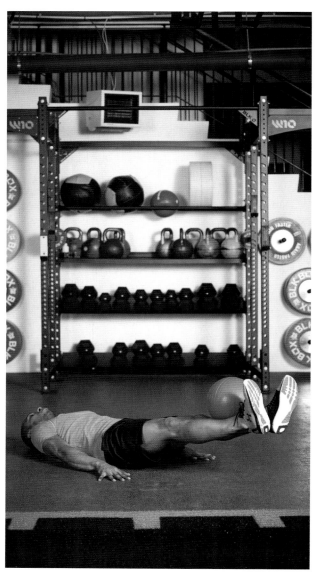

FORM Lie on your back with the ball between your ankles. Raise your legs up until they are vertical then lower them under control to the start position and repeat the exercise.

6 Standing Russian twist

REPS 12 **REST** 90sec

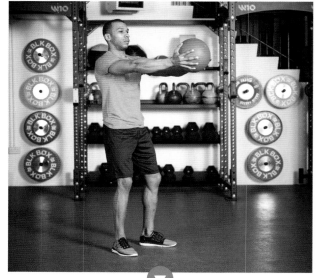

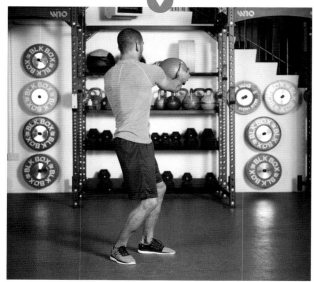

FORM Stand tall, holding the ball in both hands. Rotate to one side and then the other, keeping your abs engaged. That's one rep.

WORKOUT 2 FINISHER

Do 1 round of this finisher after you have completed all four rounds of the main circuit

Wall ball blast

CHALLENGE 50 wall throws as quickly as possible

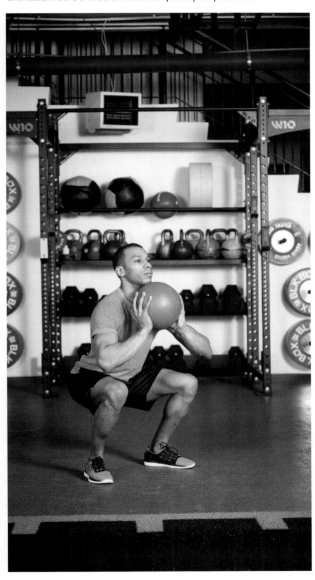

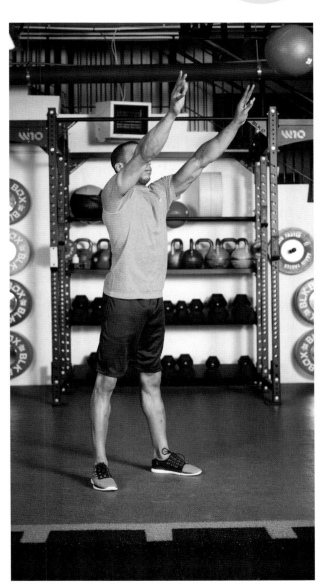

WHY This is a great test of your power endurance because you should aim to put maximum effort into each throw but, because the reps are high, you'll soon be suffering with the lactic acid build-up.

HOW Stand about one meter from a wall, go into a half squat then straighten up and throw the ball at the wall. Catch it and repeat the move, aiming to hit the same spot on the wall each time as a test of your coordination.

WORKOUT 3 BARBELL CIRCUIT

1 Deadlift

REPS 12 **REST** 10sec

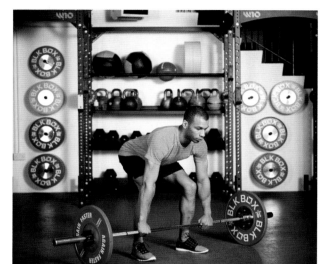

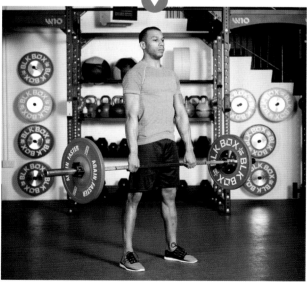

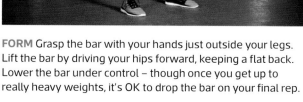

FORM Grasp the bar with your hands just outside your legs. Lift the bar by driving your hips forward, keeping a flat back. Lower the bar under control – though once you get up to really heavy weights, it's OK to drop the bar on your final rep.

2 Bent–over row

REPS 12 **REST** 10sec

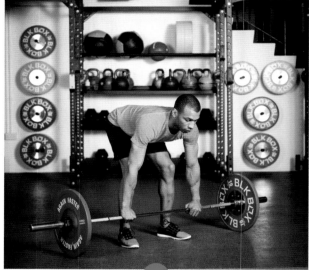

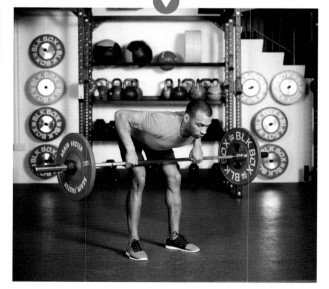

FORM Bend at the hips until you're at a roughly 45° angle to the floor. Pull the bar up to touch your belly button and then lower under control. If you're moving your upper body to shift the bar, the weight's too heavy.

3 Romanian deadlift

REPS 12 **REST** 10sec

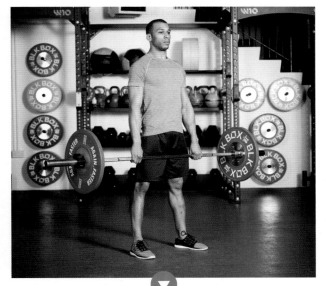

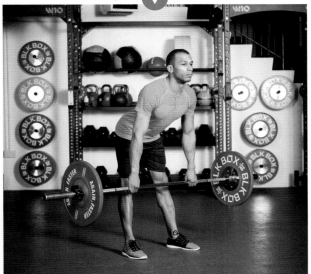

FORM Hold the bar with an overhand grip and push your backside back to send the bar down the front of your thighs. Lower until you feel a strong stretch in your hamstrings then straighten up to the start.

4 Clean

REPS 12 **REST** 10sec

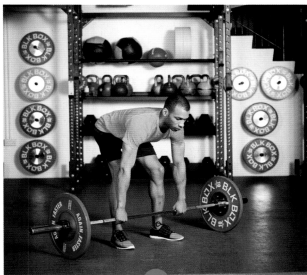

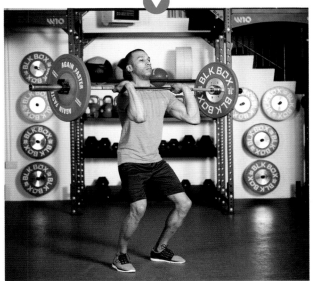

FORM Start by holding the bar with a shoulder-width grip in front of your thighs. Squat down slightly, then drive through your heels to explode upwards, using the momentum to help pull the bar up to chest height and catching it on your chest.

WORKOUT 3 BARBELL CIRCUIT

5 Front squat

REPS 12 **REST** 10sec

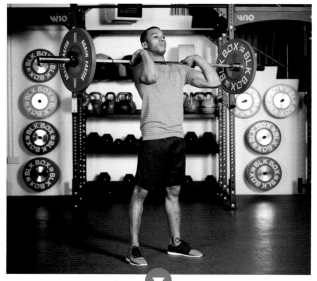

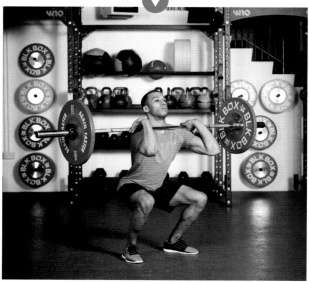

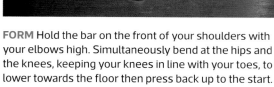

FORM Hold the bar on the front of your shoulders with your elbows high. Simultaneously bend at the hips and the knees, keeping your knees in line with your toes, to lower towards the floor then press back up to the start.

6 Overhead press

REPS 12 **REST** 90sec

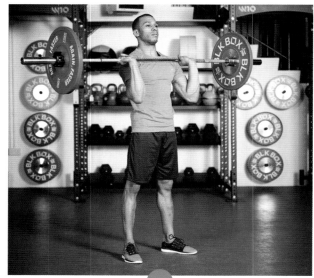

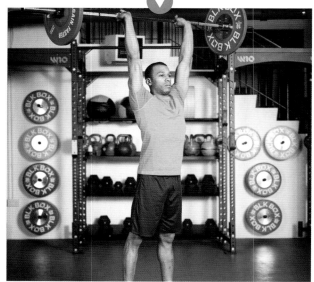

FORM With your feet shoulder-width apart, position a bar on your upper chest, gripping it with hands just wider than shoulder-width apart. Brace your abs as you press the bar straight upwards. Pause at the top, then lower.

WORKOUT 3 FINISHER

Do 1 round of this finisher after you have completed all four rounds of the main circuit

Squat death

CHALLENGE 50 squats as quickly as possible

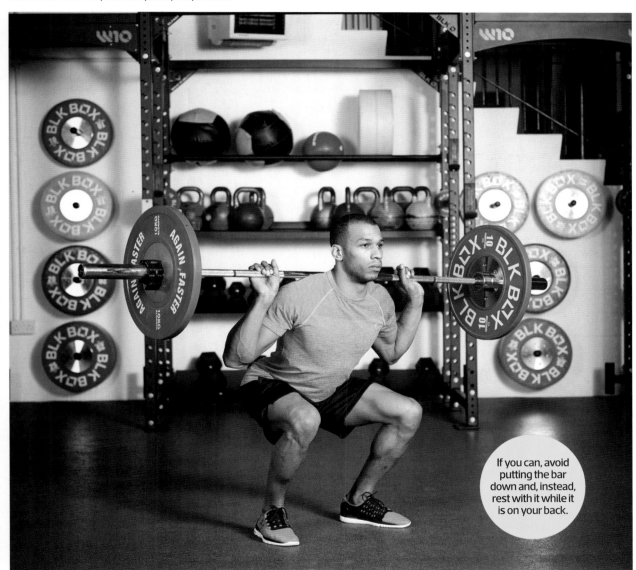

If you can, avoid putting the bar down and, instead, rest with it while it is on your back.

WHY You'll already be tired when you start this challenge so you'll quickly experience the burning sensation that signals a build up of lactic acid. It may not feel like cause for celebration but this is also great for burning fat.

HOW Perform a squat by simultaneously bending at the knees and hips to lower towards the floor, keeping your chest up and your weight on your heels and mid-foot. Aim to complete the reps in as few sets as possible.

PHASE 2

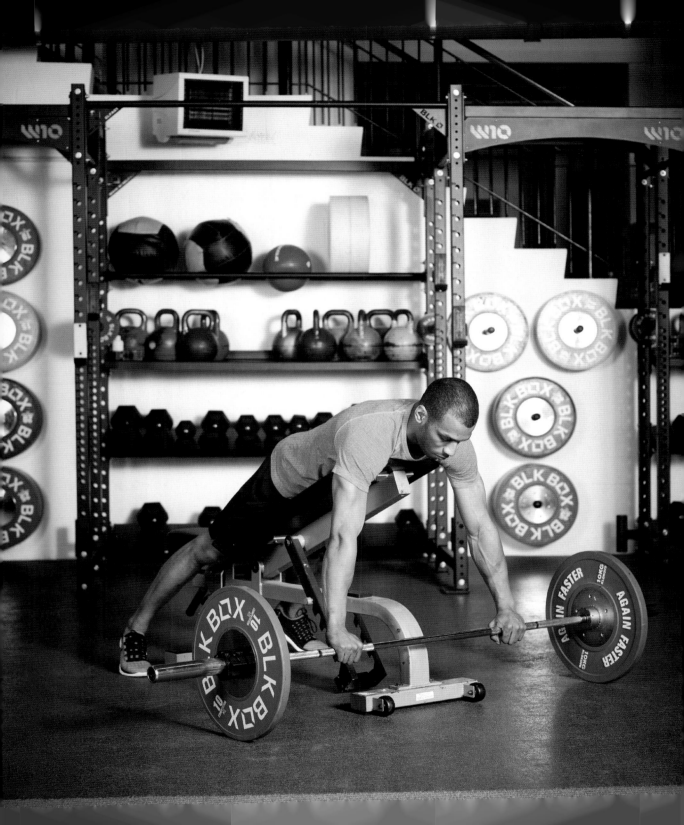

BIG FINISH

In phase two your focus moves on to building muscle

The second phase of this plan lasts for four weeks and is composed of two two-week blocks. Each week involves three workouts composed of either supersets (where you do two exercises back to back with minimal rest) or tri-sets (where you do three exercises back to back with minimal rest). The reason we've progressed from full-body circuits to supersets and tri-sets is because this shifts the emphasis away from your heart and lungs and onto your muscles. A new element for these workouts is the inclusion of tempo, which is the speed of the lift and is described using a four-digit number. The first digit is the seconds you should take to lower the weight, the second is the pause at the bottom, the third is the time you take to lift the weight and the fourth is the pause at the top.

PROGRAMME
Each workout in the first block of this second phase of the plan is made up of four supersets. The first three supersets will work every major muscle group in your body and the final superset focuses on your abs. The reason we've selected a full body workout is because it is a step forwards from the circuit plan that you followed in the first four weeks. In the second block you'll focus on specific body parts but, for now, it's a good chance to get used to a new workout structure and how that makes your muscles feel. The inclusion of supersets allows you to complete the workout in a time-efficient way because it reduces the time you spend resting. It therefore retains some of the challenge to your cardiovascular system posed by circuit training while getting you used to more advanced muscle-building strategies.

PROGRESSION
The workouts in week two involve doing the same exercises in the same order as week one. Again, that's not because we're lazy, it's because it will allow your body to take advantage of neural adaptations so you can do more reps and lift more weight. This time the progression is that you will perform two extra reps for each exercise. That may not seem like a lot but you should notice a difference. And if you're feeling really good you can increase the weight slightly. Your general aim should be to feel like you can just about complete the workout but if someone asked you to do more then you wouldn't be able to continue.

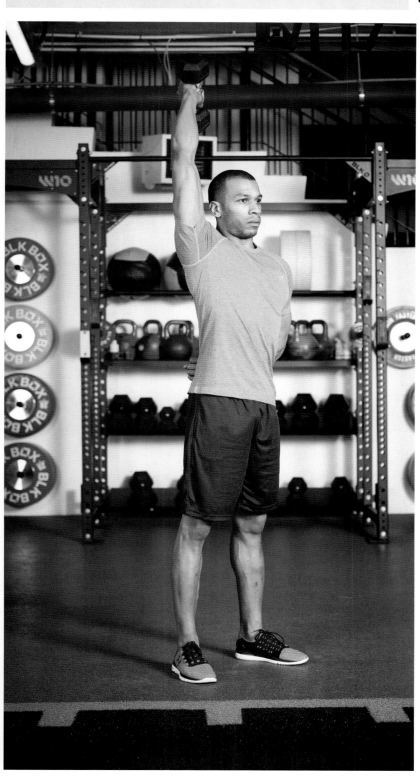

BLOCK TWO

The second fortnight of the plan uses more advanced muscle-building techniques to fine-tune your new physique. Each workout is made up of two tri-sets, each of which target a major muscle group, such as the chest or back, and an abs superset. The workouts are arranged in this way so that you do maximum damage to the muscle fibres of the target body parts which, in turn, will stimulate new muscle growth. Training just two body parts in each session, as well as your abs, is a tough way to train but, by now, you should be up to the challenge. Don't worry if you can't lift much weight by the time you get to the third exercise in a tri-set. Just focus on quality of movement and following the form guides and you'll maximise the muscle-growth benefits of the plan.

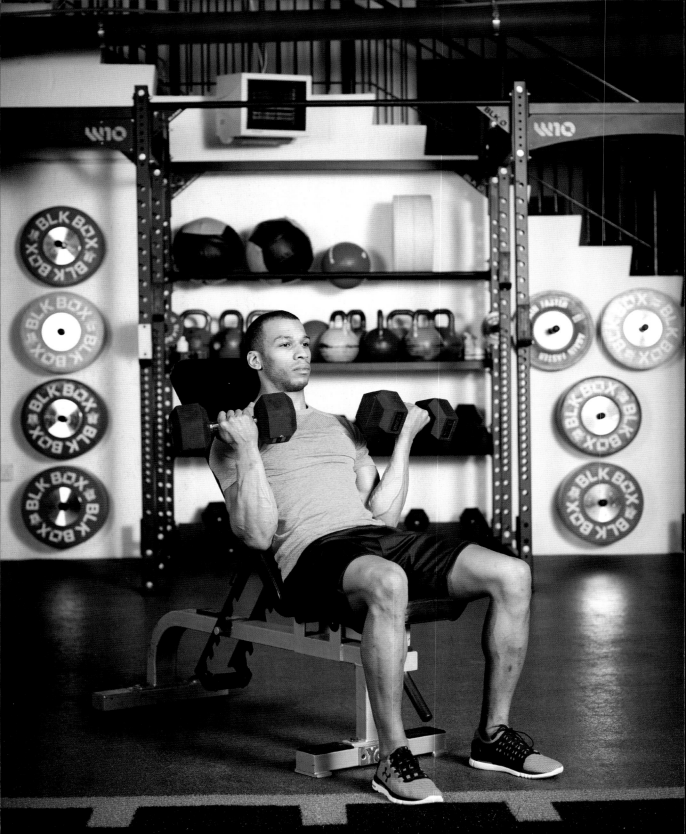

WEEK 5

MEAL PLAN

Monday

BREAKFAST
75g smoked salmon, ½ avocado, cherry tomatoes

SNACK
Post-workout shake: blend 1 scoop protein powder, 250ml milk, 1tsp butter, ½ banana and ice

LUNCH
100g quinoa mixed with chopped spring onion, crushed garlic, 1 chopped green chilli and pine nuts, served with cooked prawns

SNACK
Guacamole made with ¼ tomato, lime juice, ¼ red onion, coriander and ½ ripe avocado, served with sugar snap peas

DINNER
Chicken and cashew nut stir-fry with brown rice

SNACK
Greek yoghurt with cinnamon and a small handful of brazil nuts

Tuesday

BREAKFAST
Three scrambled eggs, spinach and a handful of mixed nuts

SNACK
50g cottage cheese with celery, carrot and cucumber sticks

LUNCH
Ham salad with ½ avocado

SNACK
100g beef jerky

DINNER
1 large cod fillet, a medium-sized serving of new potatoes and a large serving of roasted vegetables

SNACK
Greek yoghurt with cinnamon and a small handful of almonds

Wednesday

BREAKFAST
Three scrambled eggs with smoked salmon, steamed kale and ½ avocado

SNACK
Post-workout shake: blend 1 scoop protein powder, 250ml milk, 1tsp almond butter, a handful of blueberries and ice

LUNCH
Smoked salmon with spinach, cucumber and mixed salad leaves

SNACK
Guacamole made with ¼ tomato, lime juice, ¼ red onion, coriander and ½ ripe avocado, served with red pepper slices

DINNER
1 salmon fillet with brown rice, green beans and asparagus

SNACK
Whey protein mixed with 1tbsp Greek yoghurt, water and ice

Thursday

BREAKFAST
Spinach and goat's cheese three-egg omelette with a handful of almonds

SNACK
Small pot of hummus with sugar snap peas, carrots and celery

LUNCH
Roast chicken with a large baked sweet potato and broccoli

SNACK
1 apple and 25g of peanut butter

DINNER
2 homemade hamburgers (one with a wholemeal bun, one without), with a spinach and cherry tomato salad

SNACK
Greek yoghurt with cinnamon and a small handful of almonds

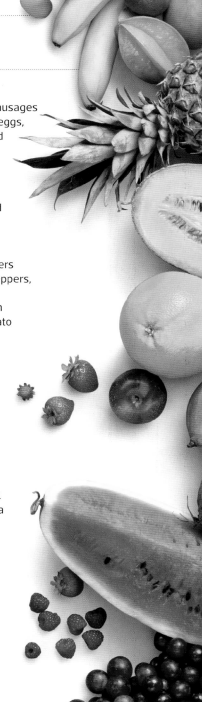

Friday

BREAKFAST
Three scrambled eggs
on brown toast

SNACK
Post-workout shake: blend
1 scoop protein powder,
230ml milk, 1tsp almond
butter, ½ banana and ice

LUNCH
Tuna and three-bean salad

SNACK
Guacamole made with
¼ tomato, lime juice, ¼
red onion, coriander and
½ ripe avocado, served
with sugar snap peas

DINNER
Grilled peppercorn ribeye
steak and Dijon butter,
served with sauteed
potatoes, grilled mushrooms
and tomatoes and steamed
green vegetables

SNACK
Greek yoghurt with
cinnamon and a small
handful of macadamia nuts

Saturday

BREAKFAST
Bacon, three scrambled
eggs, grilled mushrooms
and tomatoes

SNACK
Small pot of hummus
with celery, courgette
and cucumber sticks

LUNCH
Baked sweet potato
with goat's cheese and
spring onions, served
with a side salad

SNACK
Two boiled eggs

DINNER
Chicken stir-fry
with beansprouts and
mixed vegetables

SNACK
Greek yoghurt with
cinnamon and a small
handful of almonds

Sunday

BREAKFAST
Two grilled chicken sausages
and three scrambled eggs,
small portion of baked
beans

SNACK
50g cottage cheese
with celery, carrot and
cucumber sticks

LUNCH
Lamb grilled on skewers
with green and red peppers,
cherry tomatoes and
red onion, served with
one baked sweet potato

SNACK
1 can of tuna

DINNER
One grilled salmon
fillet with roasted
vegetables

SNACK
Greek yoghurt with
cinnamon and a small
handful of macadamia
nuts

WORKOUT 1 FULL BODY WORKOUT

1a Squat

SETS 3 **REPS** 10 **TEMPO** 4010 **REST** 10sec

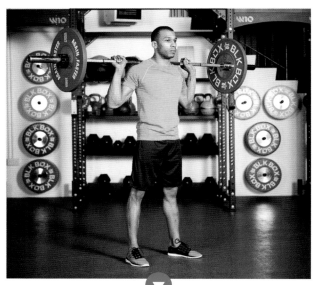

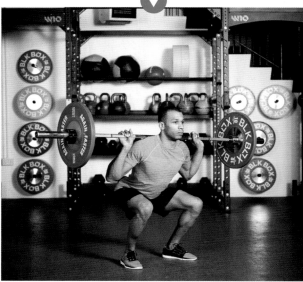

FORM Stand with your chest up and core braced. Bend your knees to squat down until your thighs are at least parallel to the ground, then push through your heels to return to the start.

1b Overhead press

SETS 3 **REPS** 10 **TEMPO** 4010 **REST** 60sec

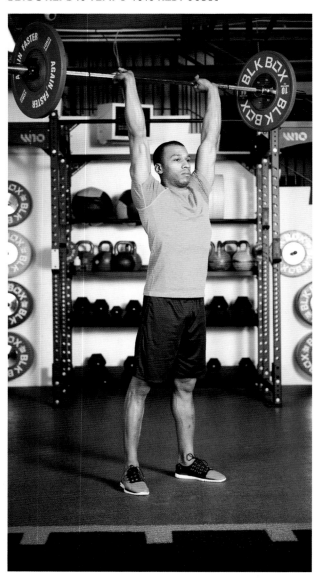

FORM Stand tall with your chest up and core braced, holding the barbell at shoulder height with palms facing forwards. Press the bar directly overhead so your arms are straight, then return slowly to the start.

2a Bench press

SETS 3 **REPS** 10 **TEMPO** 4010 **REST** 10sec

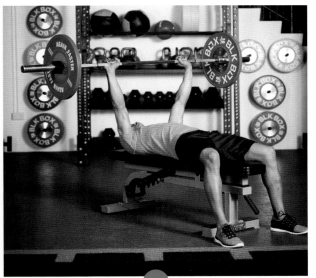

2b Bent-over row

SETS 3 **REPS** 10 **TEMPO** 4010 **REST** 60sec

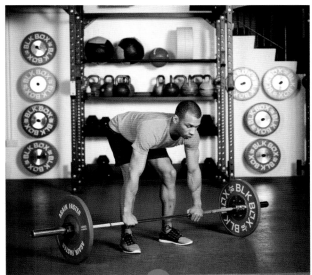

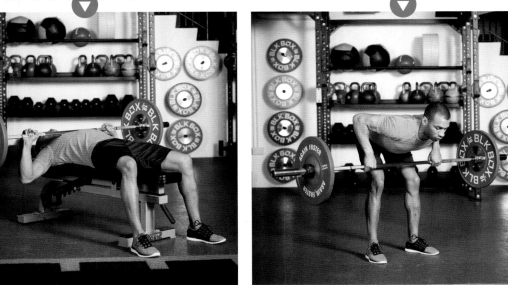

FORM Watch the ceiling, not the bar, to ensure you're pressing in the same line each time – then lower the bar to your chest, aiming to brush your T-shirt without bouncing. Press up powerfully, pause at the top, then do your next rep.

FORM Hold the bar with a shoulder-width grip, bending your knees slightly. Bend at the hips until you're at a roughly 45° angle to the floor. Pull the bar up to touch your belly button and then lower under control.

3a Biceps curl

SETS 3 **REPS** 10 **TEMPO** 4010 **REST** 10sec

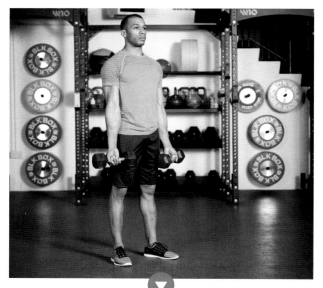

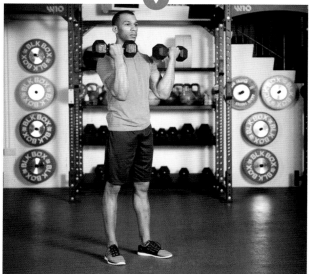

FORM Keeping your elbows tucked in to your sides, curl the dumbbells up towards your chest, stopping just before your forearms reach vertical. Lower under control to return to the start position.

3b Lying triceps extension

SETS 3 **REPS** 10 **TEMPO** 4010 **REST** 60sec

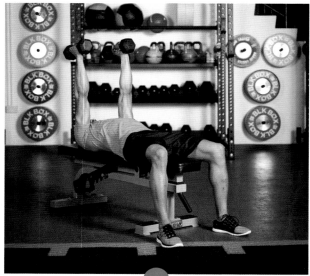

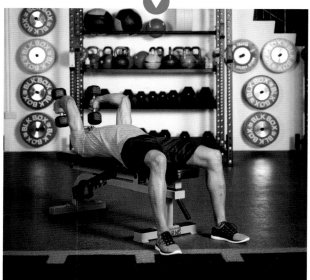

FORM Slowly lower the weights towards the top of your head by bending your elbows, keeping your upper arms as still as possible. Without arching your back, slowly return the weights to the start position by straightening your arms.

4a Mountain climber

SETS 3 **REPS** 20 **TEMPO** n/a **REST** 10sec

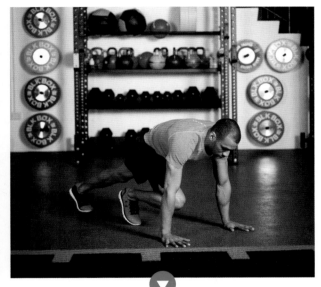

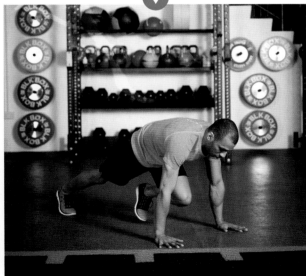

FORM Start in a position similar to a sprinter on the starting blocks. Bring one knee forwards and towards your arms, then back to the start. Repeat with the other leg, keeping the movement slow and controlled.

4b Crunch

SETS 3 **REPS** 10 **TEMPO** 4010 **REST** 60sec

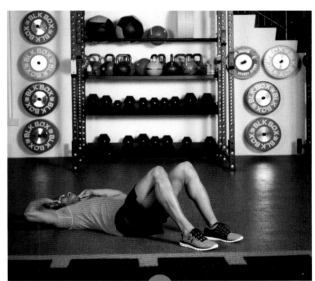

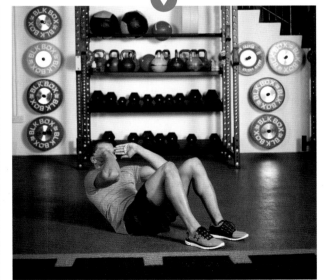

FORM Lie on your back with your knees bent and your fingers at your temples. Breathe out then contract your abs to raise your torso off the floor before lowering back down. Make sure you're not straining your neck at any point in the move.

WORKOUT 2 FULL BODY WORKOUT

1a Front squat

SETS 3 **REPS** 10 **TEMPO** 4010 **REST** 10sec

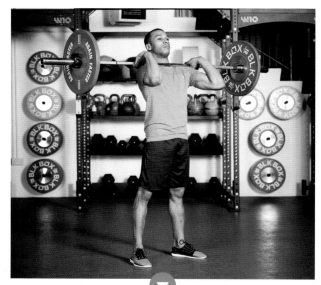

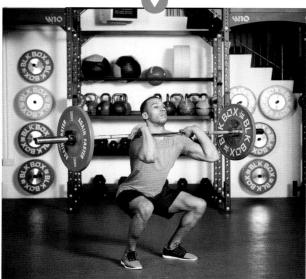

FORM Hold the bar on the front of your shoulders with your palms facing upwards. Simultaneously bend at the hips and the knees to lower towards the floor then press through your heels to stand back up again.

1b Behind neck press

SETS 3 **REPS** 10 **TEMPO** 2010 **REST** 60sec

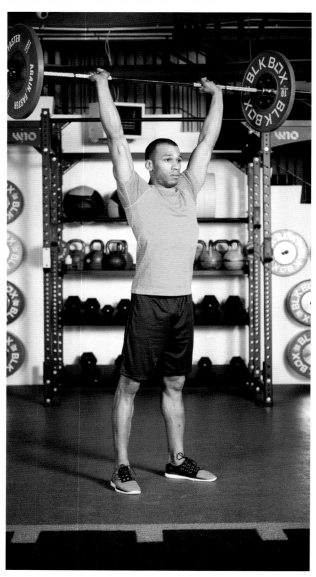

FORM Stand with the bar on your back with your hands double shoulder-width apart and your elbows pointing down. Press the weight directly up, keeping your elbows directly beneath the bar, then lower back to the start.

2a Incline bench press

SETS 3 **REPS** 10 **TEMPO** 4010 **REST** 10sec

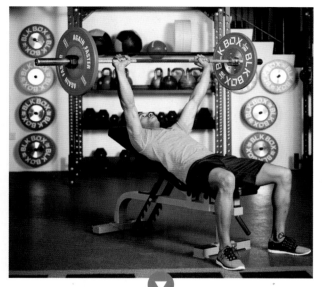

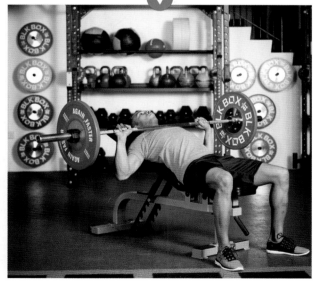

FORM Lie on a bench set at a 45° incline, holding a bar over your chest with your grip just wider than shoulder width. Lower the bar until it's touching your chest, then press it back up.

2b Prone row

SETS 3 **REPS** 10 **TEMPO** 4010 **REST** 60sec

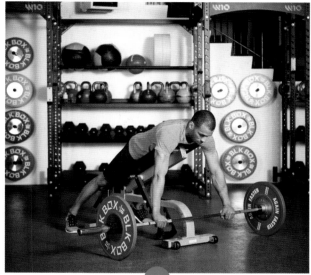

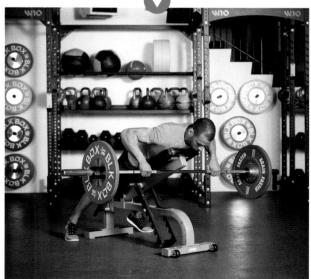

FORM Lie with your chest supported on the bench with the bar hanging straight down. Leading with your elbows, bring the bar up until it touches the bench then lower back to the start.

3a Hammer curl

SETS 3 **REPS** 10 **TEMPO** 4010 **REST** 10sec

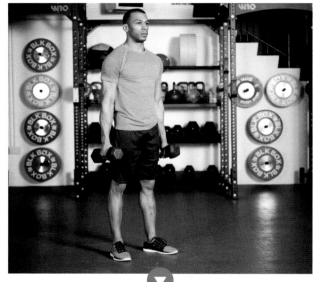

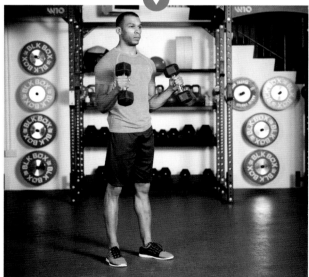

FORM With your palms facing in and your elbows tucked in to your sides, curl the dumbbells up towards your chest, stopping just before your forearms reach vertical. Lower under control to return to the start position.

3b Diamond press–up

SETS 3 **REPS** 10 **TEMPO** 2010 **REST** 60sec

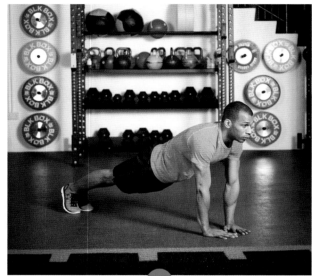

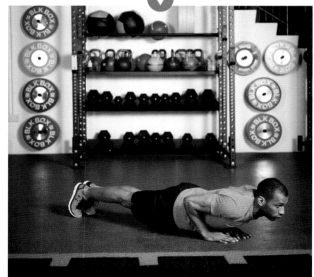

FORM Get into a press-up position, placing your hands close together so your thumbs and index fingers touch. Keeping your abs braced, lower your torso until your chest is just above the floor, and then press back up.

4a Bicycles

SETS 3 **REPS** 10 **TEMPO** n/a **REST** 10sec

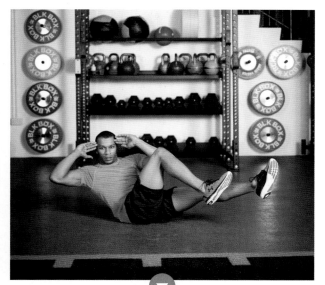

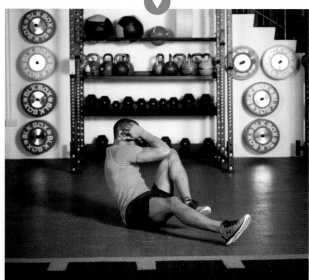

FORM Lie on the floor with your fingertips by your head and feet slightly off the floor. Bring one knee in and towards your opposite elbow, then twist to repeat the move on the other side.

4b V-sit

SETS 3 **REPS** 10 **TEMPO** 2010 **REST** 60sec

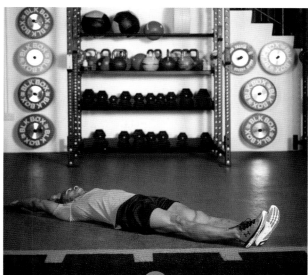

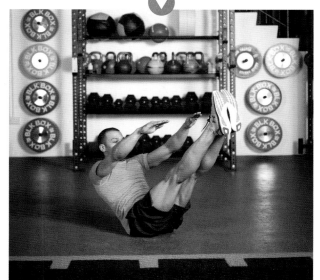

FORM Lie on your back with your arms over your head. Keeping your arms and legs straight, raise them up to meet in the middle. Pause at the top, then lower under control.

WORKOUT 3 FULL BODY WORKOUT

1a Barbell lunge

SETS 3 **REPS** 10 **TEMPO** 2010 **REST** 10sec

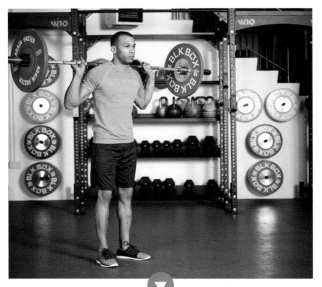

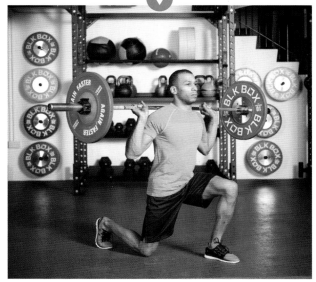

FORM With the bar on your back, take a big step forwards and lower your body until both knees are bent at 90°, then push off your front foot to return to the start position.

1b Push press

SETS 3 **REPS** 10 **TEMPO** n/a **REST** 60sec

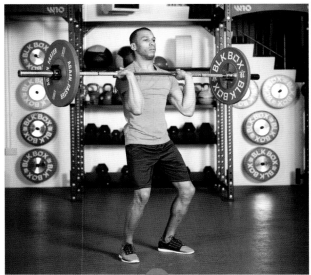

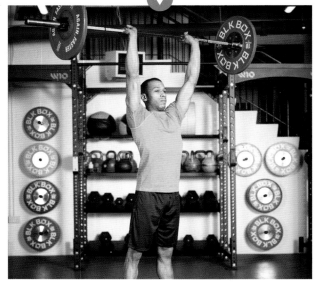

FORM Set up in the same position as the overhead press, then do a quarter-squat and press the bar overhead as explosively as possible, using the momentum to drive the bar upwards.

2a **Close-grip bench press**

SETS 3 **REPS** 10 **TEMPO** 4010 **REST** 10sec

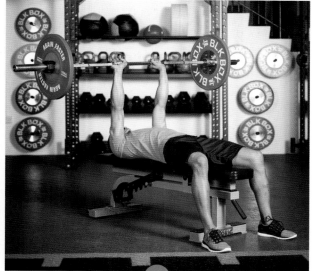

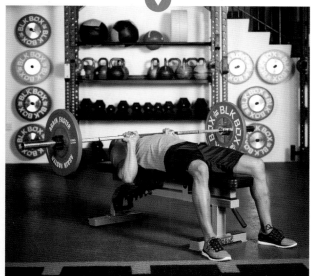

2b **Reverse-grip row**

SETS 3 **REPS** 10 **TEMPO** 4010 **REST** 60sec

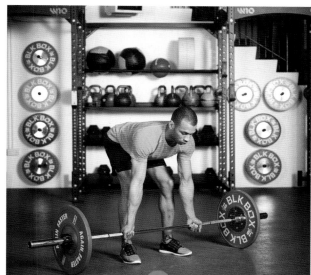

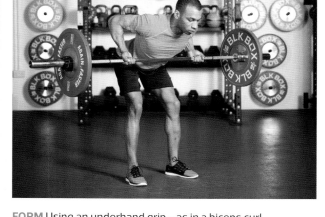

FORM Grip the bar with your hands roughly shoulder-width apart, then bring it down to your chest keeping your elbows tucked in to your sides. Pause, then press it back to the starting position.

FORM Using an underhand grip – as in a biceps curl – hold the bar with your hands at shoulder-width, bending your knees slightly. Pull the bar up to touch your belly button and then lower under control.

3a Incline biceps curl

SETS 3 **REPS** 10 **TEMPO** 4010 **REST** 10sec

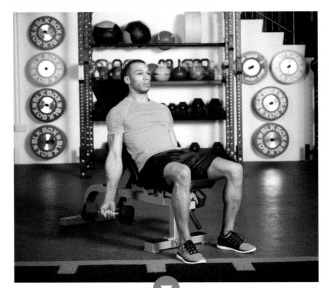

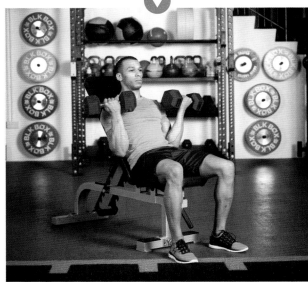

3b Overhead triceps extension

SETS 3 **REPS** 10 **TEMPO** 4010 **REST** 60sec

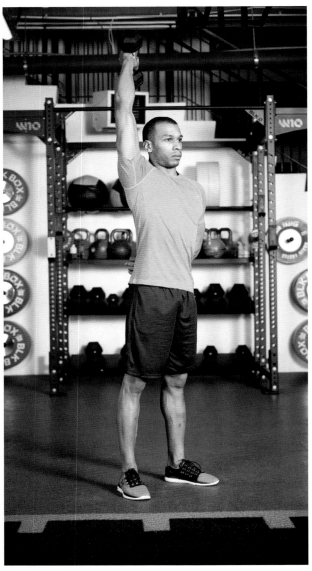

FORM Keeping your back flat against the bench and your elbows close to your sides, curl both dumbbells up to shoulder height. Squeeze your biceps at the top of the move, then slowly return the start.

FORM Stand tall, holding a dumbbell overhead in one hand. Slowly lower the dumbbell towards the back of your head by bending your elbow, keeping your upper arm as still as possible. Do five reps then switch arms.

4a Seated Russian twist

SETS 3 **REPS** 10 **TEMPO** n/a **REST** 10sec

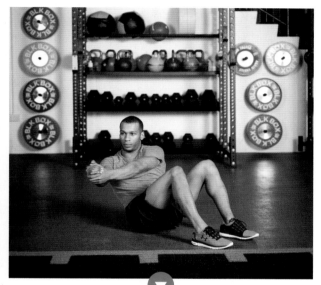

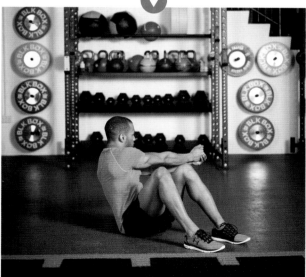

4b Leg raise

SETS 3 **REPS** 10 **TEMPO** 4010 **REST** 60sec

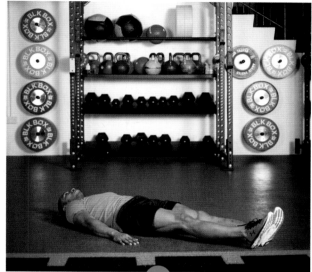

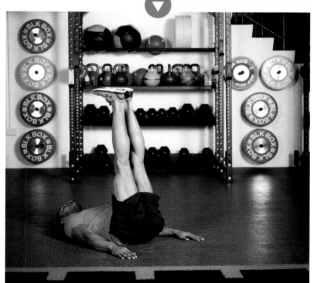

FORM Sit on the floor with your knees bent and feet flat on the floor with your hands clasped together and your arms straight. Twist to one side, pause, and then twist to the other. That's one rep.

FORM Lie on your back with your legs straight and heels slightly off the floor. Bring your legs up to a vertical position, then lower them slowly until they're just off the floor again.

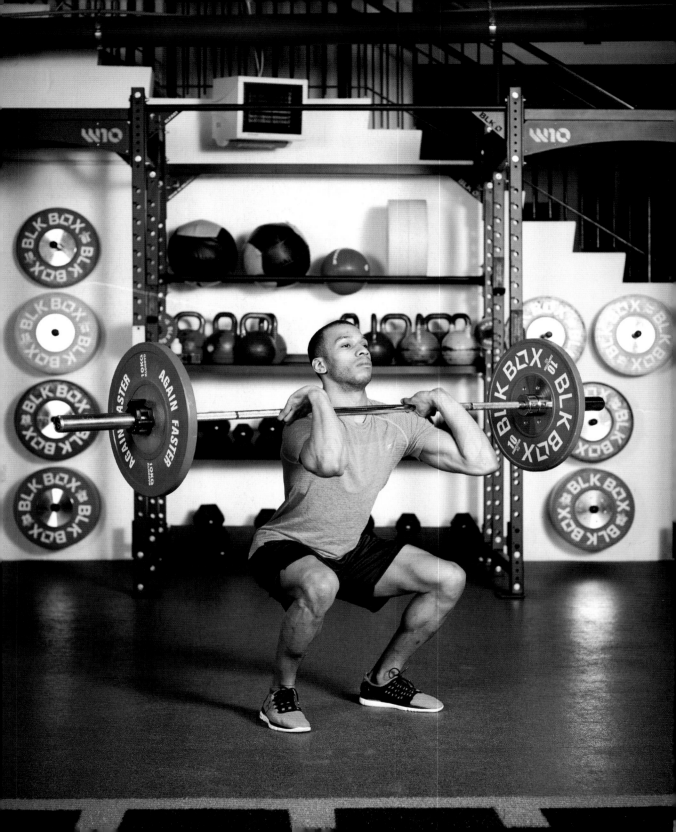

WEEK 6

MEAL PLAN

Monday

BREAKFAST
Roast chicken slices, spinach and a handful of mixed nuts

SNACK
Post-workout shake: blend 1 scoop protein powder, 200ml milk, 1tsp brazil nut butter and 1tbsp flax seeds

LUNCH
Grilled prawns with quinoa, salad, avocado and pumpkin seeds

SNACK
2 boiled eggs

DINNER
Beef meatballs in tomato sauce, with, brown rice, spinach and green vegetables

SNACK
Greek yoghurt with cinnamon and a small handful of brazil nuts

Tuesday

BREAKFAST
Three boiled eggs, ½ avocado and asparagus

SNACK
Beef slices

LUNCH
Chicken and vegetable stir-fry with broccoli, onions, green peppers and brown rice

SNACK
Guacamole and raw vegetables

DINNER
Chicken wrapped in Parma ham, with sweet potato mash and broccoli

SNACK
Greek yoghurt with cinnamon and a small handful of almonds

Wednesday

BREAKFAST
3-egg omelette with mixed peppers

SNACK
Post-workout shake: blend 1 scoop protein powder, 200ml milk, 1tsp brazil nut butter and 1tbsp flax seeds

LUNCH
2 homemade hamburgers (one with a bun and one without) with spinach salad, cherry tomatoes and chopped onion

SNACK
Guacamole and sliced red pepper

DINNER
Grilled turkey breast, with new potatoes, broccoli and mange tout

SNACK
Greek yoghurt with cinnamon and a small handful of brazil nuts

Thursday

BREAKFAST
Roast chicken slices, spinach and a handful of mixed nuts

SNACK
Ham and ½ avocado

LUNCH
Tuna salad, served with 1 baked sweet potato

SNACK
Greek yoghurt

DINNER
Steak with sauteed potatoes and roasted vegetables

SNACK
50g cottage cheese with ½ punnet blueberries and 1tbsp pumpkin seeds

Friday

BREAKFAST
Three scrambled eggs, smoked salmon and ½ avocado

SNACK
Post-workout shake: blend 1 scoop protein powder, 200ml milk, 1tsp brazil nut butter and 1tbsp flax seeds

LUNCH
Grilled prawns with salad, avocado, quinoa and pumpkin seeds

SNACK
Guacamole and sliced red pepper

DINNER
Cod fillet with new potatoes, asparagus and green beans; 1 glass red wine

SNACK
Greek yoghurt with cinnamon and a small handful of brazil nuts

Saturday

BREAKFAST
Three scrambled eggs, ½ can reduced salt and sugar beans, tomatoes, mushrooms and three rashers grilled bacon

SNACK
1tbsp peanut butter and an apple

LUNCH
Chicken and vegetable stir-fry with broccoli, onions, green peppers and brown rice

SNACK
1 can tuna

DINNER
2 homemade hamburgers with spinach salad, cherry tomatoes and chopped onion

SNACK
Whey protein mixed with 1tbsp Greek yoghurt, water and ice

Sunday

BREAKFAST
2 poached eggs, ½ an avocado mashed on two slices of toasted sourdough bread, tomatoes

SNACK
Smoked salmon and ½ avocado

LUNCH
Beef stir-fry

SNACK
1tbsp peanut butter and a banana

DINNER
Roast chicken, with new potatoes, broccoli, carrots, cabbage and gravy

SNACK
Whey protein mixed with 1tbsp Greek yoghurt, water and ice

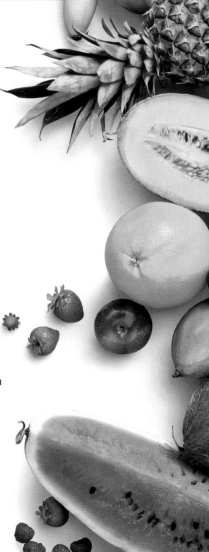

WORKOUT 1 FULL BODY WORKOUT

1a Squat

SETS 3 **REPS** 12 **TEMPO** 4010 **REST** 10sec

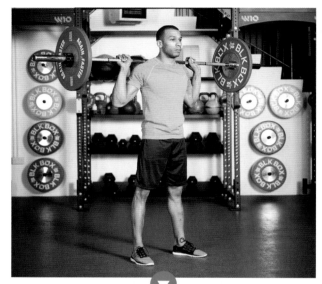

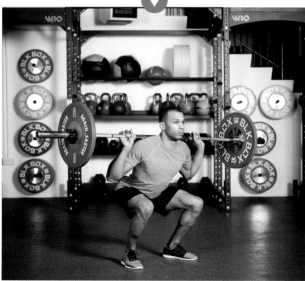

FORM Stand with your chest up and core braced. Bend your knees to squat down until your thighs are at least parallel to the ground, then push through your heels to return to the start.

1b Overhead press

SETS 3 **REPS** 12 **TEMPO** 4010 **REST** 60sec

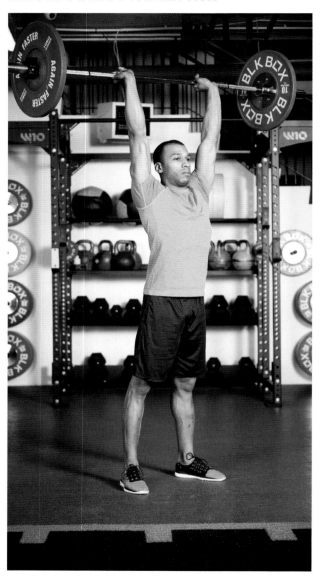

FORM Stand tall with your chest up and core braced, holding the barbell at shoulder height with palms facing forwards. Press the bar directly overhead so your arms are straight, then return slowly to the start.

2a Bench press

SETS 3 **REPS** 12 **TEMPO** 4010 **REST** 10sec

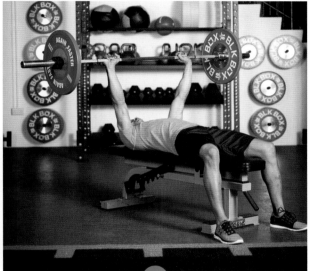

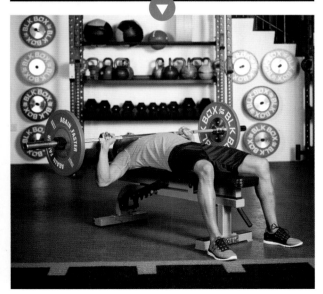

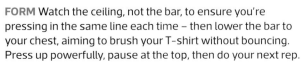

FORM Watch the ceiling, not the bar, to ensure you're pressing in the same line each time – then lower the bar to your chest, aiming to brush your T-shirt without bouncing. Press up powerfully, pause at the top, then do your next rep.

2b Bent-over row

SETS 3 **REPS** 12 **TEMPO** 4010 **REST** 60sec

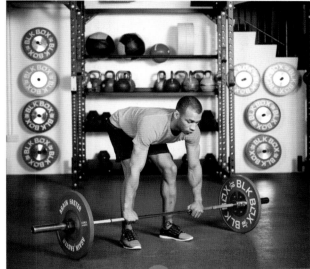

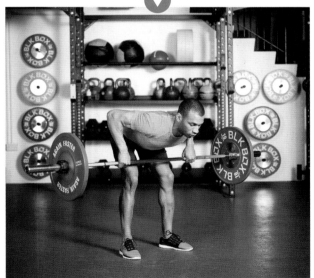

FORM Hold the bar with a shoulder-width grip, bending your knees slightly. Bend at the hips until you're at a roughly 45° angle to the floor. Pull the bar up to touch your belly button and then lower under control.

3a Biceps curl

SETS 3 **REPS** 12 **TEMPO** 4010 **REST** 10sec

3b Lying triceps extension

SETS 3 **REPS** 12 **TEMPO** 4010 **REST** 60sec

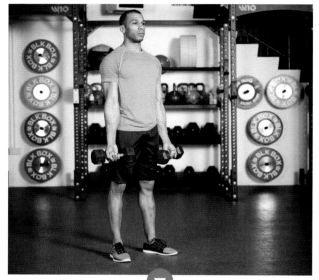

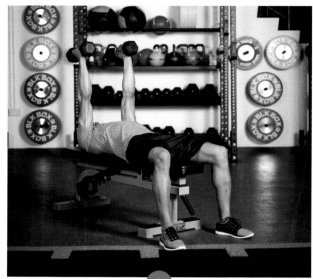

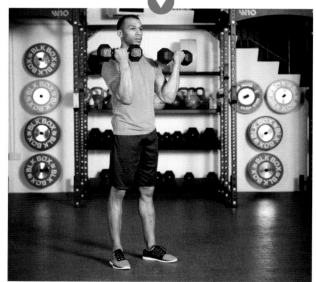

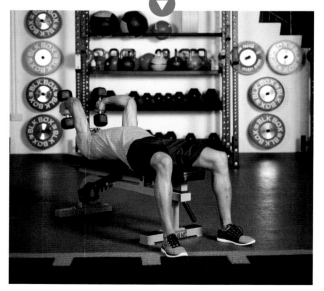

FORM Keeping your elbows tucked in to your sides, curl the dumbbells up towards your chest, stopping just before your forearms reach vertical. Lower under control to return to the start position.

FORM Slowly lower the weights towards the top of your head by bending your elbows, keeping your upper arms as still as possible. Without arching your back, slowly return the weights to the start position by straightening your arms.

4a Mountain climber

SETS 3 **REPS** 20 **TEMPO** n/a **REST** 10sec

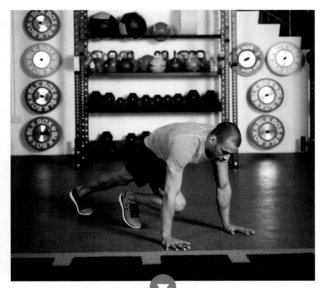

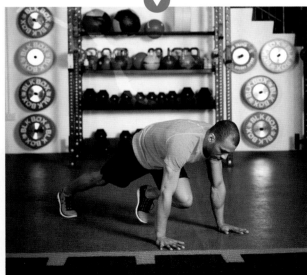

FORM Start in a position similar to a sprinter on the starting blocks. Bring one knee forwards and towards your arms, then back to the start. Repeat with the other leg, keeping the movement slow and controlled.

4b Crunch

SETS 3 **REPS** 12 **TEMPO** 4010 **REST** 60sec

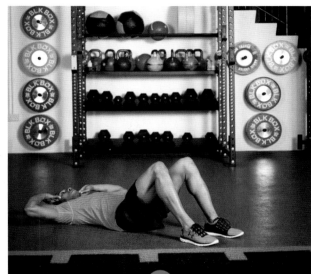

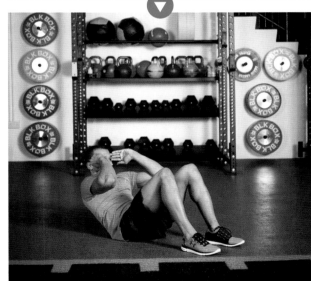

FORM Lie on your back with your knees bent and your fingers at your temples. Breathe out then contract your abs to raise your torso off the floor before lowering back down. Make sure you're not straining your neck at any point in the move.

WORKOUT 2 FULL BODY WORKOUT

1a Front squat

SETS 3 REPS 12 TEMPO 4010 REST 10sec

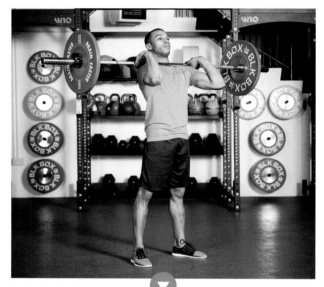

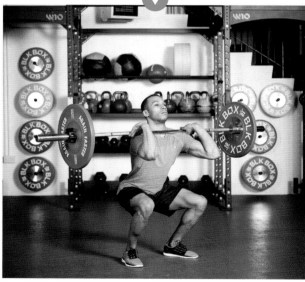

FORM Hold the bar on the front of your shoulders with your palms facing upwards. Simultaneously bend at the hips and the knees to lower towards the floor then press through your heels to stand back up again.

1b Behind neck press

SETS 3 REPS 12 TEMPO 2010 REST 60sec

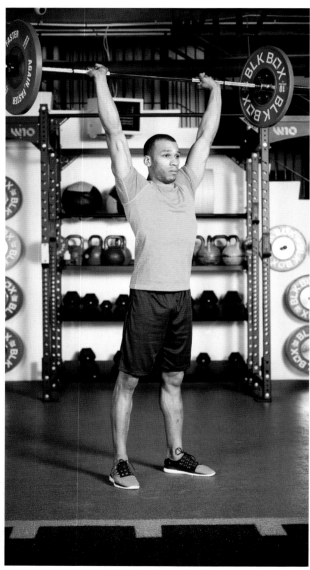

FORM Stand with the bar on your back with your hands double shoulder-width apart and your elbows pointing down. Press the weight directly up, keeping your elbows directly beneath the bar, then lower back to the start.

LOSE YOUR BELLY FOR GOOD!

2a Incline bench press

SETS 3 **REPS** 12 **TEMPO** 4010 **REST** 10sec

2b Prone row

SETS 3 **REPS** 12 **TEMPO** 4010 **REST** 60sec

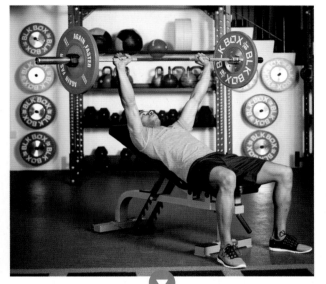

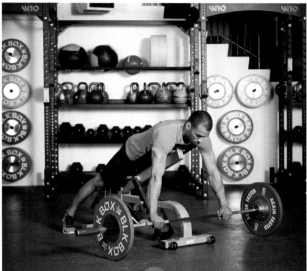

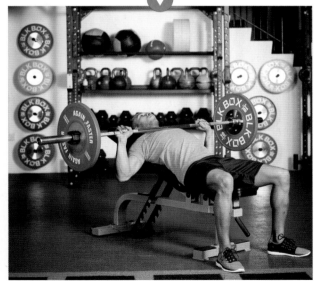

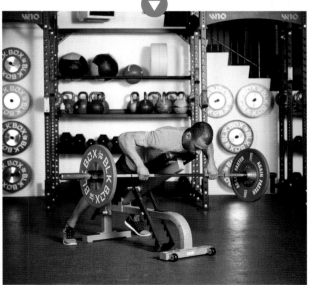

FORM Lie on a bench set at a 45° incline, holding a bar over your chest with your grip just wider than shoulder width. Lower the bar until it's touching your chest, then press it back up.

FORM Lie with your chest supported on the bench with the bar hanging straight down. Leading with your elbows, bring the bar up until it touches the bench then lower back to the start.

3a Hammer curl

SETS 3 **REPS** 12 **TEMPO** 4010 **REST** 10sec

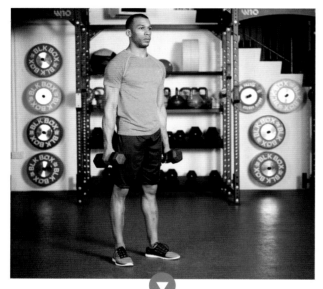

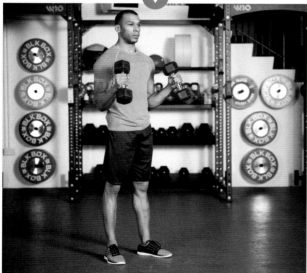

FORM With your palms facing in and your elbows tucked in to your sides, curl the dumbbells up towards your chest, stopping just before your forearms reach vertical. Lower under control to return to the start position.

3b Diamond press–up

SETS 3 **REPS** 12 **TEMPO** 2010 **REST** 60sec

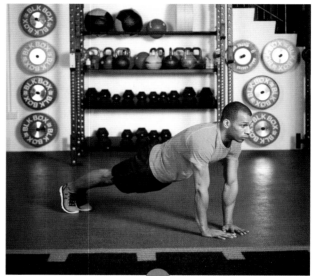

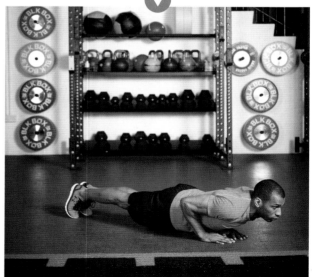

FORM Get into a press–up position, placing your hands close together so your thumbs and index fingers touch. Keeping your abs braced, lower your torso until your chest is just above the floor, and then press back up.

4a Bicycles

SETS 3 **REPS** 12 **TEMPO** n/a **REST** 10sec

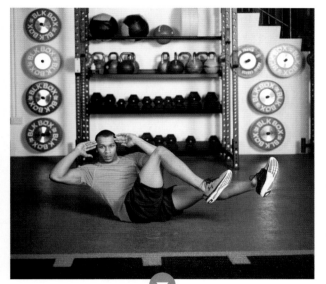

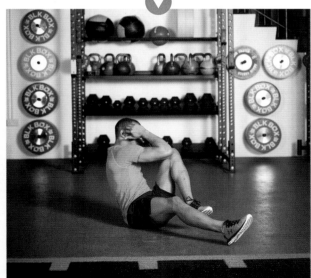

4b V-sit

SETS 3 **REPS** 12 **TEMPO** 2010 **REST** 60sec

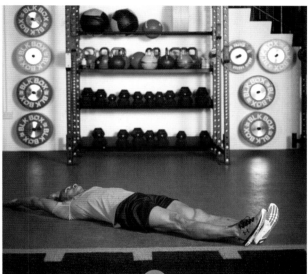

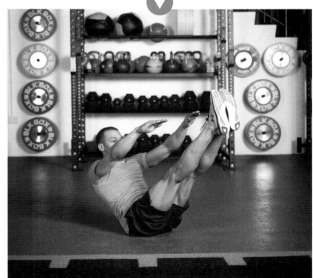

FORM Lie on the floor with your fingertips by your head and feet slightly off the floor. Bring one knee in and towards your opposite elbow, then twist to repeat the move on the other side.

FORM Lie on your back with your arms over your head. Keeping your arms and legs straight, raise them up to meet in the middle. Pause at the top, then lower under control.

WORKOUT 3 FULL BODY WORKOUT

1a Barbell lunge

SETS 3 **REPS** 12 **TEMPO** 2010 **REST** 10sec

1b Push press

SETS 3 **REPS** 12 **TEMPO** n/a **REST** 60sec

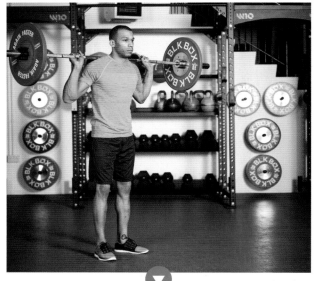

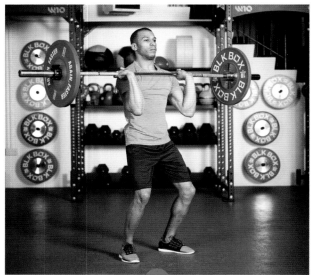

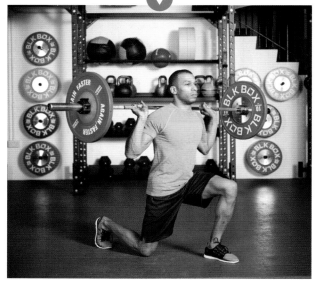

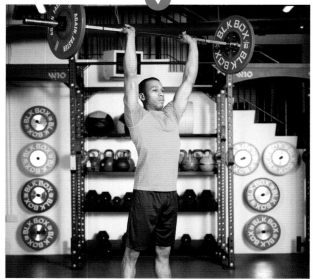

FORM With the bar on your back, take a big step forwards and lower your body until both knees are bent at 90°, then push off your front foot to return to the start position.

FORM Set up in the same position as the overhead press, then do a quarter-squat and press the bar overhead as explosively as possible, using the momentum to drive the bar upwards.

2a Close-grip bench press

SETS 3 REPS 12 TEMPO 4010 REST 10sec

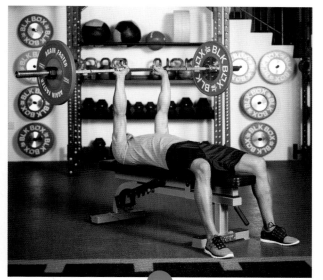

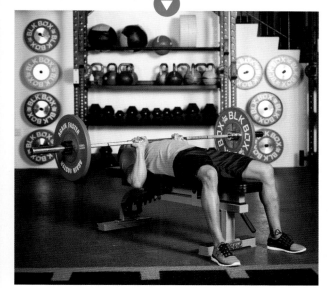

FORM Grip the bar with your hands roughly shoulder-width apart, then bring it down to your chest keeping your elbows tucked in to your sides. Pause, then press it back to the starting position.

2b Reverse-grip row

SETS 3 REPS 12 TEMPO 4010 REST 60sec

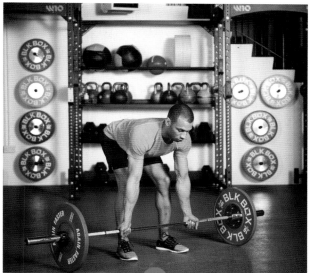

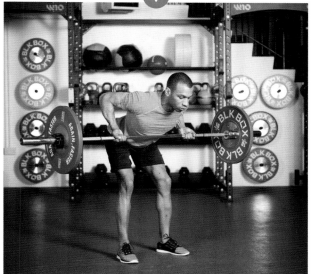

FORM Using an underhand grip - as in a biceps curl - hold the bar with your hands at shoulder-width, bending your knees slightly. Pull the bar up to touch your belly button and then lower under control.

3a Incline biceps curl

SETS 3 **REPS** 12 **TEMPO** 4010 **REST** 10sec

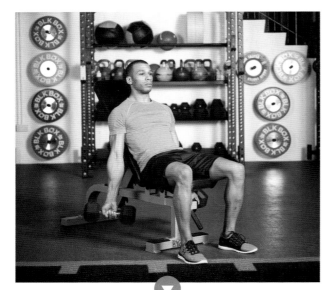

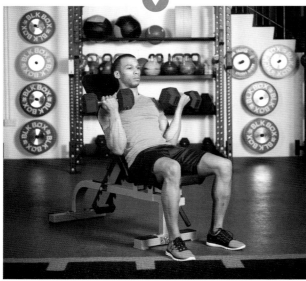

3b Overhead triceps extension

SETS 3 **REPS** 12 **TEMPO** 4010 **REST** 60sec

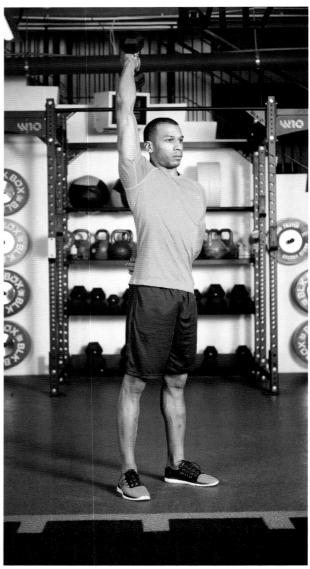

FORM Keeping your back flat against the bench and your elbows close to your sides, curl both dumbbells up to shoulder height. Squeeze your biceps at the top of the move, then slowly return the start.

FORM Stand tall, holding a dumbbell overhead in one hand. Slowly lower the dumbbell towards the back of your head by bending your elbow, keeping your upper arm as still as possible. Do five reps then switch arms.

4a Seated Russian twist

SETS 3 **REPS** 12 **TEMPO** n/a **REST** 10sec

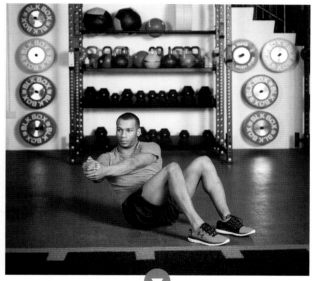

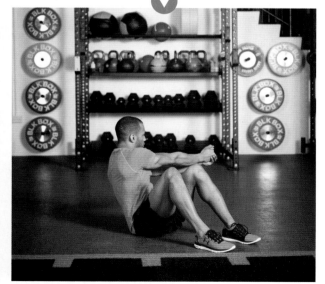

FORM Sit on the floor with your knees bent and feet flat on the floor with your hands clasped together and your arms straight. Twist to one side, pause, and then twist to the other. That's one rep.

4b Leg raise

SETS 3 **REPS** 12 **TEMPO** 4010 **REST** 60sec

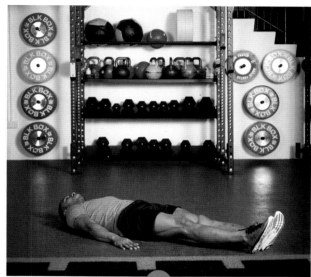

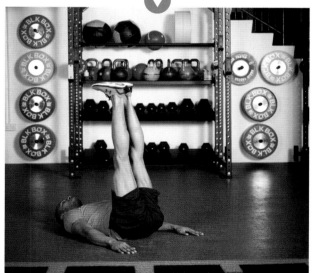

FORM Lie on your back with your legs straight and heels slightly off the floor. Bring your legs up to a vertical position, then lower them slowly until they're just off the floor again.

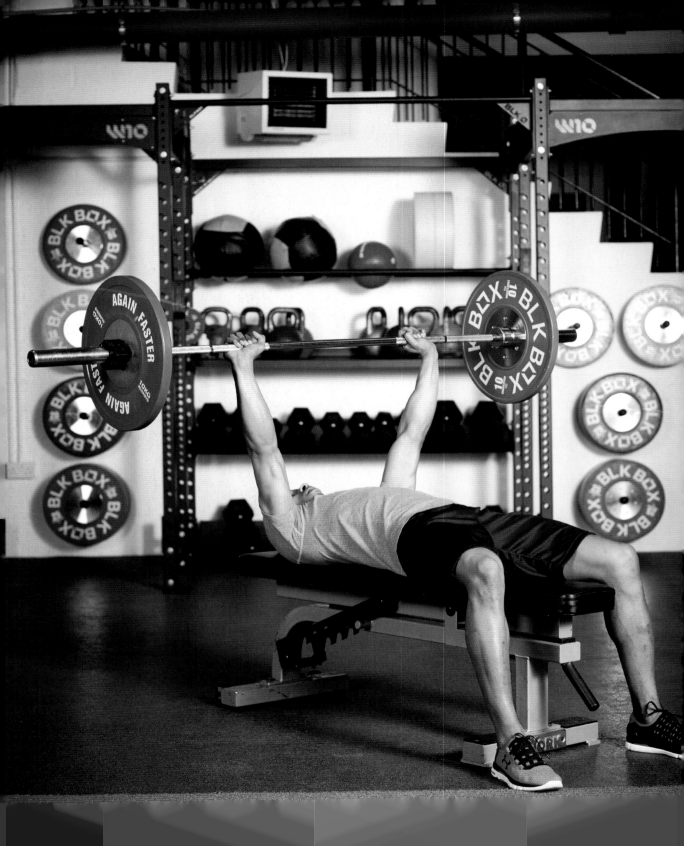

WEEK 7

MEAL PLAN

Monday

BREAKFAST
Roast chicken slices
with a bowl of grapes
and melon cubes

SNACK
Post-workout shake: blend 1
scoop protein powder, 100ml
milk, 1/2 banana, 75ml semi-
skimmed milk and 1tbsp oats

LUNCH
One large sweet potato
with 1 can tuna in water
(drained) and spinach

SNACK
Small pot of hummus
with celery, carrot and
cucumber sticks

DINNER
Ginger chicken stir-fry
with onion, pepper, mange
tout and brown rice

SNACK
Greek yoghurt with
cinnamon and a small
handful of pecan nuts

Tuesday

BREAKFAST
Three scrambled eggs,
spinach and a handful
of mixed nuts

SNACK
Celery sticks, brazil nut
butter and 10 raisins

LUNCH
Grilled prawns with a wild
rice mixed salad, 1/2 avocado
and pumpkin seeds

SNACK
100g beef jerky

DINNER
Chilli beef with brown
rice and grated cheese

SNACK
Greek yoghurt with
cinnamon and a small
handful of walnuts

Wednesday

BREAKFAST
2 poached eggs, smoked
salmon, steamed spinach
and 1/2 avocado

SNACK
Post-workout shake: blend
1 scoop protein powder, 1/2
banana, raspberries, 150ml
skimmed milk, 100ml natural
yoghurt, 1tbsp sunflower
seeds and 20g rolled oats

LUNCH
Lamb steak with new
potatoes, a side salad
and cherry tomatoes

SNACK
Small pot of hummus
with celery, carrot and
cucumber sticks

DINNER
1 cod fillet with sweet potato
and steamed vegetables

SNACK
Greek yoghurt with
cinnamon and a small
handful of pecan nuts

Thursday

BREAKFAST
Spinach and goat's cheese
three-egg omelette and
a handful of almonds

SNACK
Celery sticks and
brazil nut butter

LUNCH
Grilled prawns, quinoa,
mixed salad, 1/2 avocado
and pumpkin seeds

SNACK
2 scrambled eggs
and spinach

DINNER
Tuna steak, new potatoes,
asparagus, broccoli
and cauliflower

SNACK
Greek yoghurt with
cinnamon and a small
handful of walnuts

Friday

BREAKFAST
150g porridge oats cooked with 200ml semi-skimmed milk, ½ banana and 1tsp honey; stir in ½ scoop whey protein at the end

SNACK
Post-workout shake: blend 1 scoop protein powder, 100ml milk, ½ banana, 75ml semi-skimmed milk and 1tbsp oats

LUNCH
Ham and avocado salad

SNACK
Small pot of hummus with celery, carrot and cucumber sticks

DINNER
2 pork chops with sweet potato mash and green beans; 1 glass red wine

SNACK
Greek yoghurt with cinnamon and a small handful of pecan nuts

Saturday

BREAKFAST
Three scrambled eggs, two grilled sausages, grilled mushrooms and tomatoes

SNACK
Celery sticks with almond butter

LUNCH
100g quinoa mixed with 2 boiled eggs, 1 chicken breast and broccoli

SNACK
1 can of tuna

DINNER
Homemade beef chilli with brown rice and grated cheese

SNACK
Greek yoghurt with cinnamon and a small handful of walnuts

Sunday

BREAKFAST
2 poached eggs on sourdough toast and smoked salmon

SNACK
A handful of brazil nuts

LUNCH
Diced lamb grilled on skewers with diced green and red peppers, diced onion and cherry tomatoes, with 1 baked sweet potato

SNACK
Ham and ½ avocado

DINNER
Grilled chicken breast with brown rice and a beetroot, spinach and goat's cheese salad

SNACK
Greek yoghurt with cinnamon and a small handful of walnuts

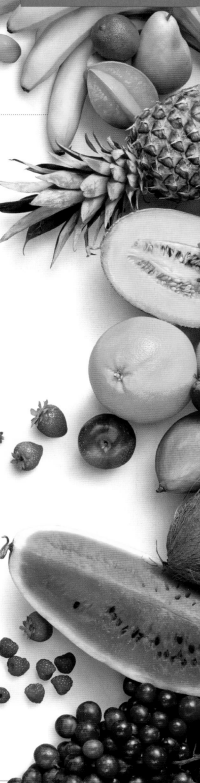

WORKOUT 1 CHEST, BACK AND ABS

1a Bench press

SETS 3 **REPS** 10 **TEMPO** 4010 **REST** 10sec

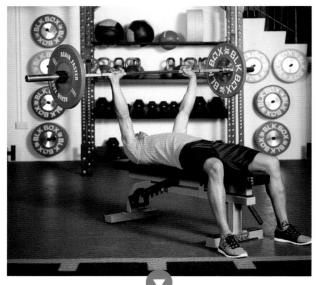

1b Dumbbell flye

SETS 3 **REPS** 10 **TEMPO** 4010 **REST** 10sec

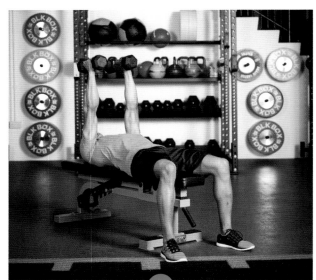

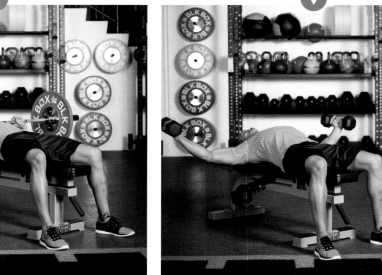

FORM Watch the ceiling, not the bar, to ensure you're pressing in the same line each time – then lower the bar to your chest, aiming to brush your T-shirt without bouncing. Press up powerfully, pause at the top, then do your next rep.

FORM Keeping a slight bend in your elbows, slowly lower the weights to the sides as far as is comfortable, feeling the stretch in your chest. Squeeze your chest to reverse the movement and raise the weights back to the top.

1c Press-up

SETS 3 **REPS** 10 **TEMPO** 4010 **REST** 60sec

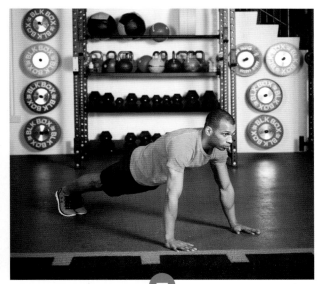

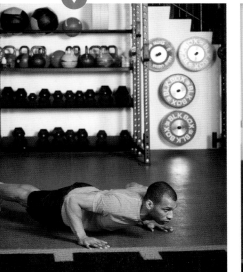

FORM Get into a press-up position with your hands just outside shoulder width apart. Keeping your abs braced, lower your body until your chest touches the floor - keeping your thighs off it - and then press up.

2a Bent-over row

SETS 3 **REPS** 10 **TEMPO** 4010 **REST** 10sec

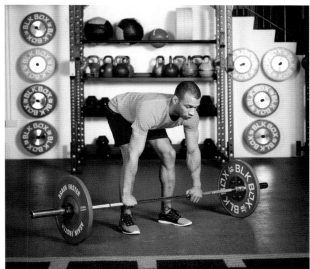

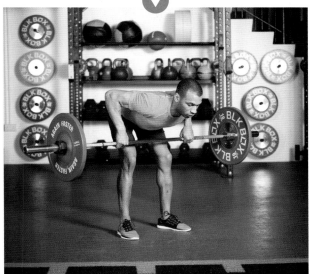

FORM Hold the bar with a shoulder-width grip, bending your knees slightly. Bend at the hips until you're at a roughly 45° angle to the floor. Pull the bar up to touch your belly button and then lower under control.

2b Reverse flye

SETS 3 **REPS** 10 **TEMPO** 4010 **REST** 10sec

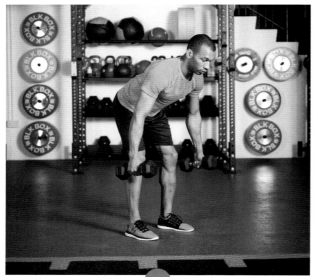

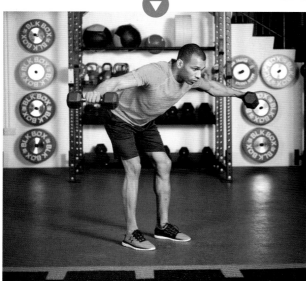

FORM Leaning forwards at the hips with a weight in each hand, keep your back flat and bring the weights upwards as if you were spreading your wings, aiming to bring your shoulder blades together at the top of the move.

2c Dumbbell row

SETS 3 **REPS** 10 **TEMPO** 4010 **REST** 60sec

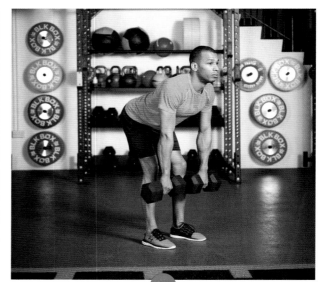

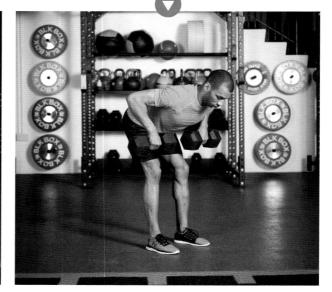

FORM Stand with your back straight and your shoulder blades retracted, holding a set of dumbbells, then bend your knees slightly and lean forwards from the hips. Pull the dumbbells up to just below chest level. Pause, then lower under control.

3a Gym ball crunch

SETS 3 **REPS** 10 **TEMPO** 3010 **REST** 10sec

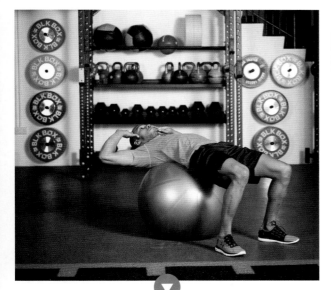

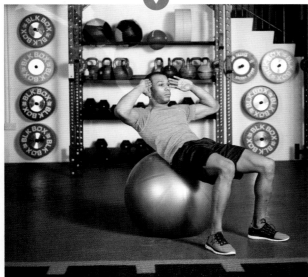

3b Gym ball decline plank

SETS 3 **TIME** 30secs **REST** 60sec

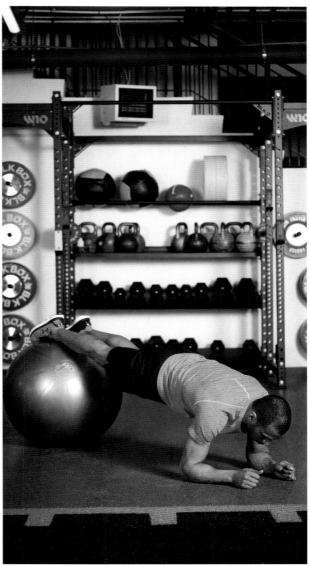

FORM Lie over a gym ball with feet flat on the floor and fingers touching your temples. Contract your abs to raise your torso up off the ball, pause at the top, then lower back to the start.

FORM Hold your body in a straight line from head to heels with your elbows directly beneath your shoulders and both feet on a gym ball. Brace your abs to hold this position without letting your hips sag.

WORKOUT 2 SHOULDERS, LEGS AND ABS

1a Cuban press

SETS 3 **REPS** 10 **TEMPO** n/a **REST** 10sec

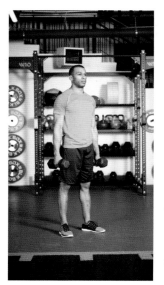
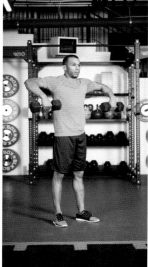

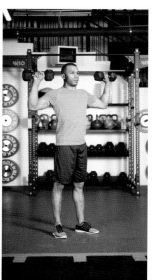
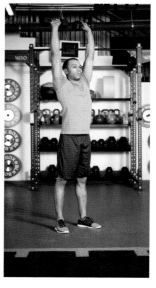

FORM Raise your arms to the sides until your elbows are bent at 90°. Keeping your upper arms horizontal, rotate your elbows until your hands point up. Press the weights directly overhead. Reverse the movement back to the start.

1b Overhead press

SETS 3 **REPS** 10 **TEMPO** 4010 **REST** 10sec

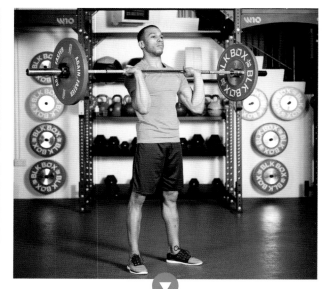

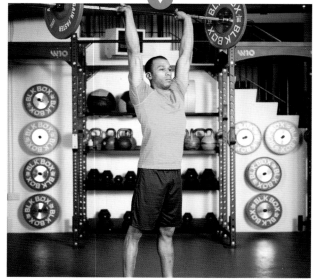

FORM Stand tall with your chest up and core braced, holding the barbell at shoulder height with palms facing forwards. Press the bar directly overhead so your arms are straight, then return slowly to the start.

1c Lateral raise

SETS 3 **REPS** 10 **TEMPO** 4010 **REST** 60sec

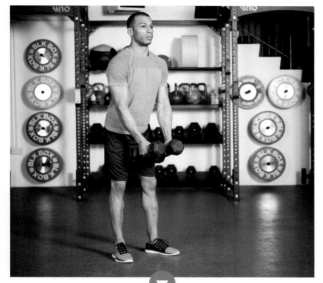

2a Front squat

SETS 3 **REPS** 10 **TEMPO** 4010 **REST** 10sec

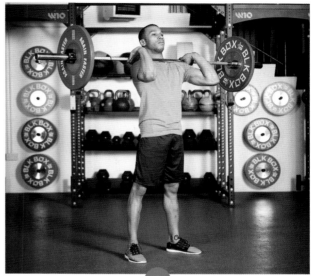

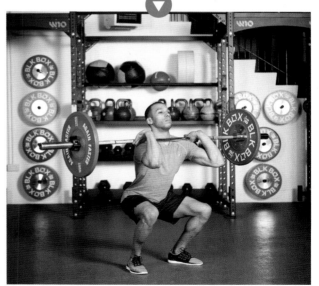

FORM Hold a light dumbbell in each hand by your sides with your palms facing one another. Keeping a slight bend in your elbows, raise the weights out to the sides making sure you use your muscles and not momentum.

FORM Hold the bar on the front of your shoulders with your palms facing upwards. Simultaneously bend at the hips and the knees to lower towards the floor then press through your heels to stand back up again.

2b Romanian deadlift

SETS 3 **REPS** 10 **TEMPO** 4010 **REST** 10sec

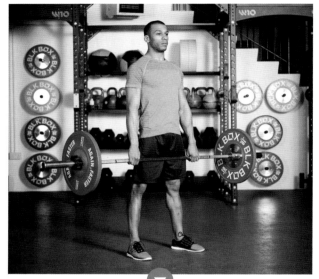

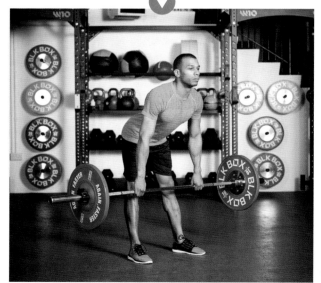

FORM Keeping a slight bend in your knees, bend forwards from the hips and lower the bar down the front of your shins until you feel a good stretch in your hamstrings. Reverse the move back to the start by pushing your hips forwards.

2c Mountain climber

SETS 3 **REPS** 10 **TEMPO** n/a **REST** 60sec

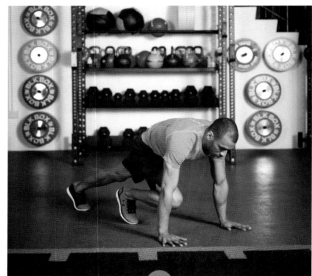

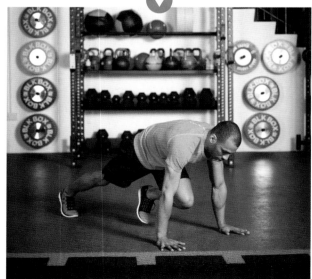

FORM Start in a position similar to a sprinter on the starting blocks. Bring one knee forwards and towards your arms, then back to the start. Repeat with the other leg, keeping the movement slow and controlled.

3a Gym ball crunch twist

SETS 3 **REPS** 12 **TEMPO** 3010 **REST** 10sec

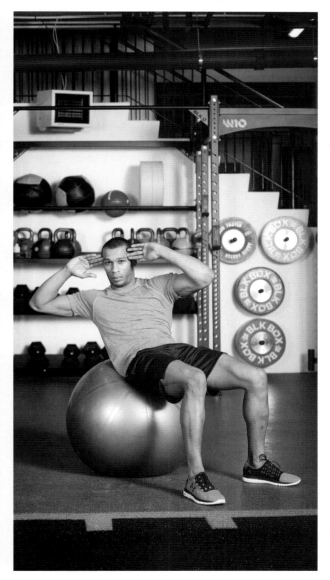

FORM Lie over a Swiss ball with feet flat on the floor and fingers touching your temples. Contract your abs to raise your torso up off the ball, then rotate to one side. Pause at the top, lower back to the start, then repeat to the other side.

3b Gym ball incline plank

SETS 3 **TIME** 30secs **REST** 60sec

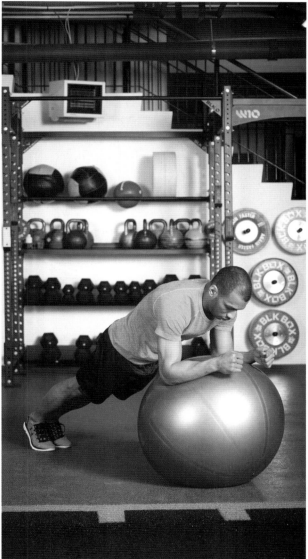

FORM Hold your body in a straight line from head to heels with your elbows on a gym ball directly beneath your shoulders. Brace your abs to hold this position without letting your hips sag.

WORKOUT 3 ARMS AND ABS

1a Incline biceps curl

SETS 3 **REPS** 10 **TEMPO** 4010 **REST** 10sec

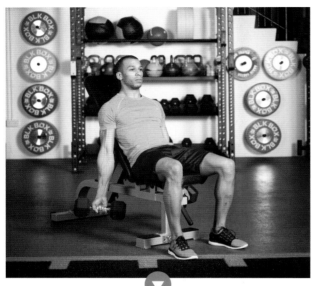

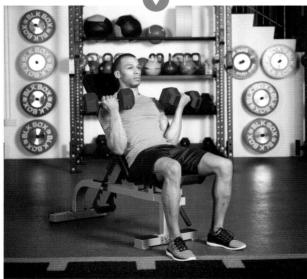

FORM Keeping your back flat against the bench and your elbows close to your sides, curl both dumbbells up to shoulder height. Squeeze your biceps at the top of the move, then slowly return the start.

1b Hammer curl

SETS 3 **REPS** 10 **TEMPO** 4010 **REST** 10sec

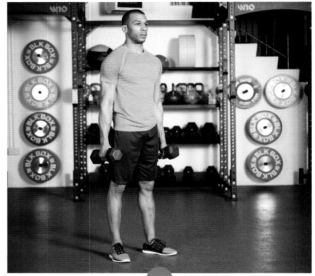

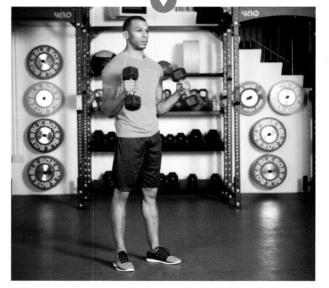

FORM With your palms facing in and your elbows tucked in to your sides, curl the dumbbells up towards your chest, squeezing your biceps at the top. Lower under control to return to the start position.

1c Alternating biceps curl

SETS 3 **REPS** 10 **TEMPO** 4010 **REST** 60sec

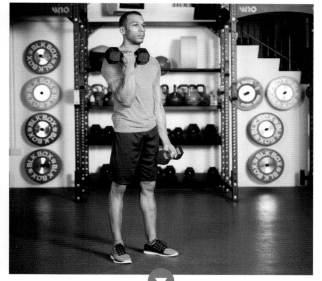

FORM Hold a pair of dumbbells with your palms facing forwards. Keeping your elbows tucked in to your sides, curl one dumbbell up towards your chest, then lower it and raise the other.

2a Lying triceps extension

SETS 3 **REPS** 10 **TEMPO** 4010 **REST** 10sec

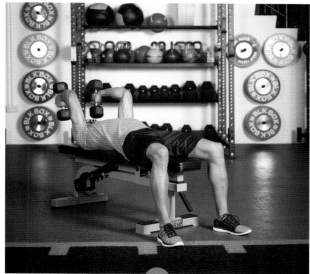

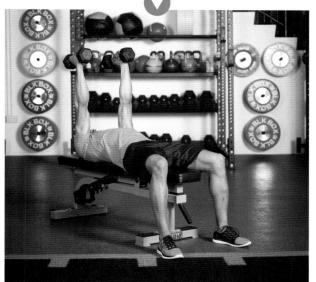

FORM Slowly lower the weights towards the top of your head by bending your elbows, keeping your upper arms as still as possible. Without arching your back, slowly return the weights to the start position by straightening your arms.

2b Bench dip

SETS 3 **REPS** 10 **TEMPO** 4010 **REST** 10sec

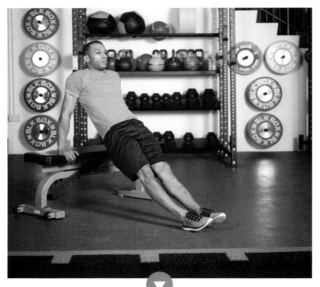

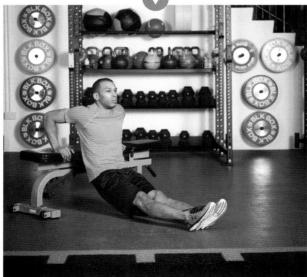

FORM Place your palms on a bench with your legs straight and out in front of you. Bend at the elbows to lower towards the floor, ensuring that your elbows don't flare outwards, then press back up to the start.

2c Eccentric diamond press-up

SETS 3 **REPS** 10 **TEMPO** 4010 **REST** 60sec

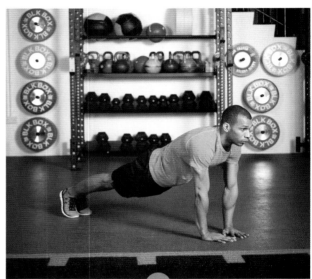

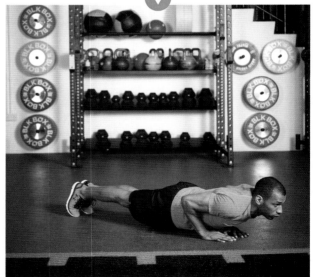

FORM Placing your hands close together so your thumbs and index fingers touch, lower your torso until your chest is just above the floor then go onto your knees to get back to the start and repeat the move.

3a Gym ball crunch

SETS 3 **REPS** 10 **TEMPO** 3010 **REST** 10sec

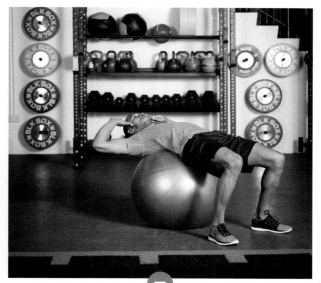

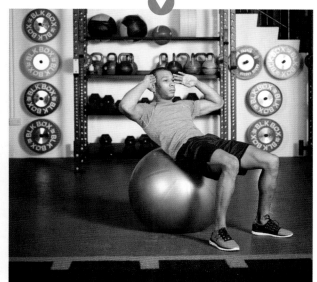

FORM Lie over a Swiss ball with feet flat on the floor and fingers touching your temples. Contract your upper abs to raise your torso up off the ball, pause at the top, then lower back to the start.

3b Gym ball rollout

SETS 3 **REPS** 10 **TEMPO** 4010 **REST** 60sec

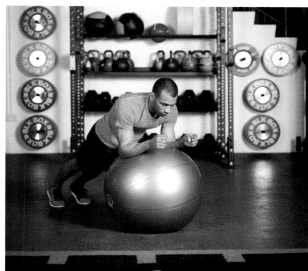

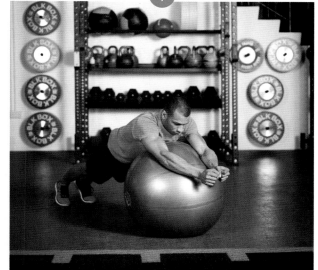

FORM Kneel in front of a Swiss ball with both elbows resting on arm. Keeping your core braced, roll the ball away from your knees until your body forms a straight line from head to hips. Pause, then reverse the movement back to the start.

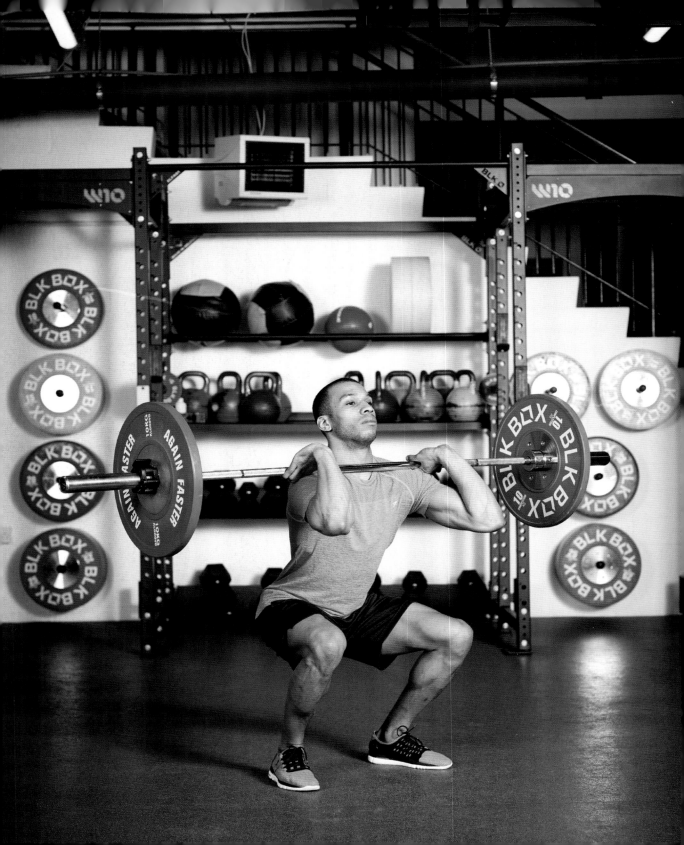

WEEK 8

MEAL PLAN

Monday

BREAKFAST
Spinach and goat's cheese three-egg omelette with a handful of almonds

SNACK
Post-workout shake: blend 150ml milk, 1 scoop chocolate whey protein powder, ½ banana and 2tbsp Greek yoghurt

LUNCH
Salmon fillet, 150g couscous and 150g Greek salad with sundried tomatoes, cucumber, red onion, feta cheese, olives, ½ chilli and 1 pepper

SNACK
Hummus, 1 carrot, 100g sliced green and red pepper

DINNER
Grilled chicken breast with brown rice chilli sauce and roasted vegetables

SNACK
100g cottage cheese and 2 wholegrain rice cakes

Tuesday

BREAKFAST
Roast beef slices with wilted spinach and asparagus

SNACK
Pineapple slices and cottage cheese

LUNCH
Grilled chicken breast with a wholemeal wrap, mixed salad and ½ avocado

SNACK
1 banana and a handful of almonds

DINNER
120g tuna steak, brown rice stir-fried broccoli, green beans and spinach

SNACK
Greek yoghurt and blueberries

Wednesday

BREAKFAST
2 boiled eggs and 1 slice rye bread

SNACK
Post-workout shake: blend 150ml milk, 1 scoop chocolate whey protein powder, ½ banana and 2tbsp Greek yoghurt

LUNCH
200g can tuna mixed with 2tsp chickpeas, lettuce, cucumber, spring onion, carrot, coriander, 30g (dry weight) cooked brown rice, olive oil and balsamic vinegar

SNACK
Apple and a handful of pumpkin seeds

DINNER
120g salmon, new potatoes, stir-fried broccoli, green beans, red pepper and spinach

SNACK
100g cottage cheese and 2 wholegrain rice cakes

Thursday

BREAKFAST
Three grilled sausages and three scrambled eggs

SNACK
Pineapple slices and cottage cheese

LUNCH
One carton carrot and coriander soup with steamed green vegetables

SNACK
1 banana and a handful of almonds

DINNER
Large chicken salad with toasted walnuts

SNACK
Greek yoghurt with cinnamon and brazil nuts

Friday

BREAKFAST
Roast chicken slices
and a handful of nuts

SNACK
Post-workout shake:
blend 150ml milk,
1 scoop chocolate whey
protein powder, ½ banana
and 2tbsp Greek yoghurt

LUNCH
Ham and avocado salad

SNACK
A handful of almonds, raisins
and dark chocolate chips

DINNER
Beef fajitas: 200g fillet
steak cut into strips with
1 red, 1 green pepper
and 2 tortilla wraps

SNACK
100g cottage cheese and
2 wholegrain rice cakes

Saturday

BREAKFAST
Three scrambled eggs,
½ can reduced salt and
sugar beans, tomatoes,
mushrooms and 2
rashers grilled bacon

SNACK
Pineapple slices and
cottage cheese

LUNCH
Tuna salad with cherry
tomatoes and beetroot

SNACK
1 banana and a handful
of almonds

DINNER
200g salmon teriyaki with
brown rice, spinach and
steamed courgette slices

SNACK
Greek yoghurt with
cinnamon and brazil nuts

Sunday

BREAKFAST
Three grilled chicken
sausages and three
scrambled eggs,
small portion of
baked beans

SNACK
A handful of almonds
and raisins

LUNCH
One carton of carrot
and coriander soup
with steamed
green vegetables

SNACK
Hummus with carrot
sticks and 100g sliced
green and red peppers

DINNER
Roast beef, sweet
potato mash, carrots,
spinach, broccoli
and parsnips

SNACK
100g cottage cheese
on 2 wholegrain
rice cakes

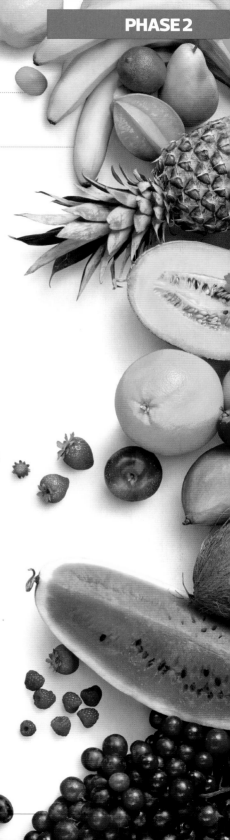

WORKOUT 1 CHEST, BACK AND ABS

1a Bench press

SETS 3 **REPS** 12 **TEMPO** 4010 **REST** 10sec

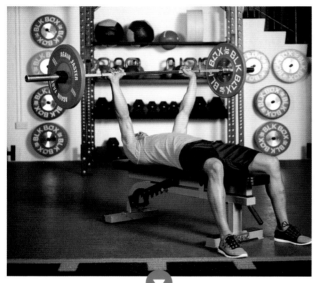

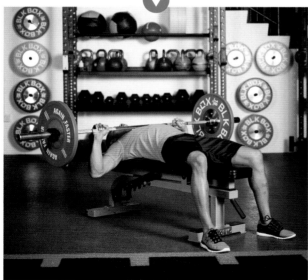

FORM Watch the ceiling, not the bar, to ensure you're pressing in the same line each time – then lower the bar to your chest, aiming to brush your T-shirt without bouncing. Press up powerfully, pause at the top, then do your next rep.

1b Dumbbell flye

SETS 3 **REPS** 12 **TEMPO** 4010 **REST** 10sec

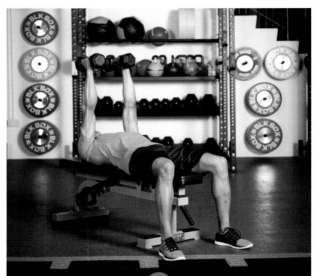

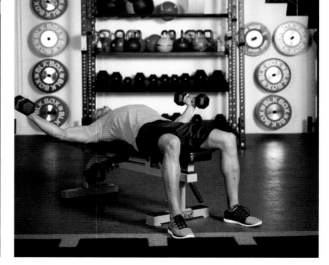

FORM Keeping a slight bend in your elbows, slowly lower the weights to the sides as far as is comfortable, feeling the stretch in your chest. Squeeze your chest to reverse the movement and raise the weights back to the top.

1c Press-up

SETS 3 **REPS** 12 **TEMPO** 4010 **REST** 60sec

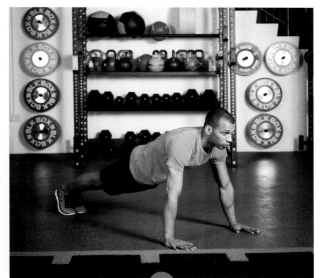

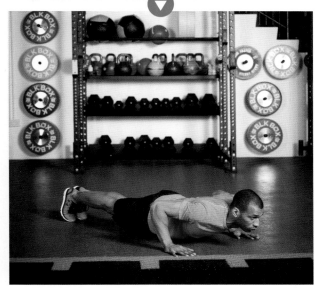

FORM Get into a press-up position with your hands just outside shoulder width apart. Keeping your abs braced, lower your body until your chest touches the floor – keeping your thighs off it – and then press up.

2a Bent-over row

SETS 3 **REPS** 12 **TEMPO** 4010 **REST** 10sec

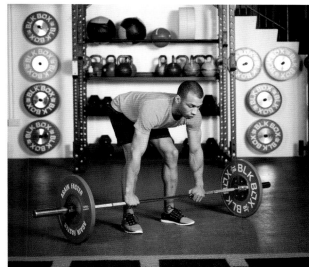

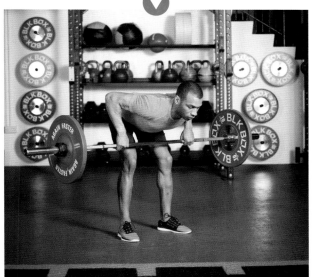

FORM Hold the bar with a shoulder-width grip, bending your knees slightly. Bend at the hips until you're at a roughly 45° angle to the floor. Pull the bar up to touch your belly button and then lower under control.

2b Reverse flye

SETS 3 **REPS** 12 **TEMPO** 4010 **REST** 10sec

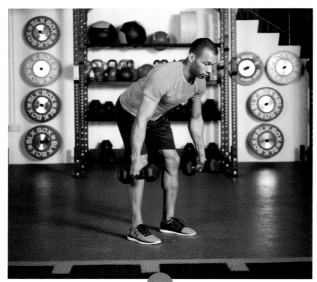

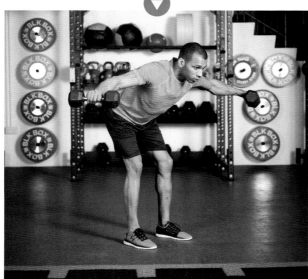

FORM Leaning forwards at the hips with a weight in each hand, keep your back flat and bring the weights upwards as if you were spreading your wings, aiming to bring your shoulder blades together at the top of the move.

2c Dumbbell row

SETS 3 **REPS** 12 **TEMPO** 4010 **REST** 60sec

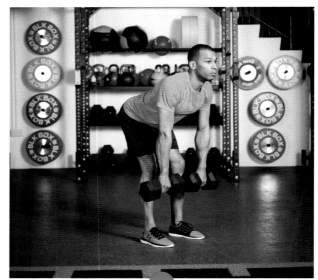

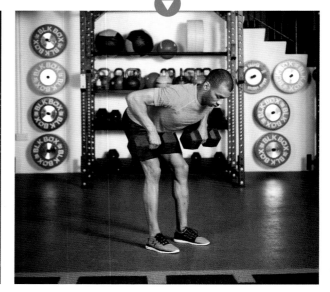

FORM Stand with your back straight and your shoulder blades retracted, holding a set of dumbbells, then bend your knees slightly and lean forwards from the hips. Pull the dumbbells up to just below chest level. Pause, then lower under control.

3a Gym ball crunch

SETS 3 **REPS** 12 **TEMPO** 3010 **REST** 10sec

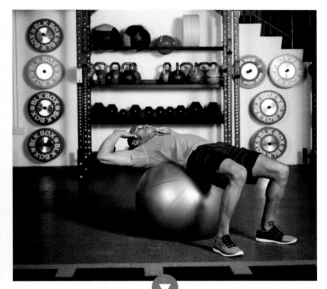

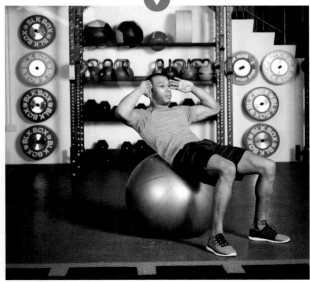

3b Gym ball decline plank

SETS 3 **TIME** 40secs **REST** 60sec

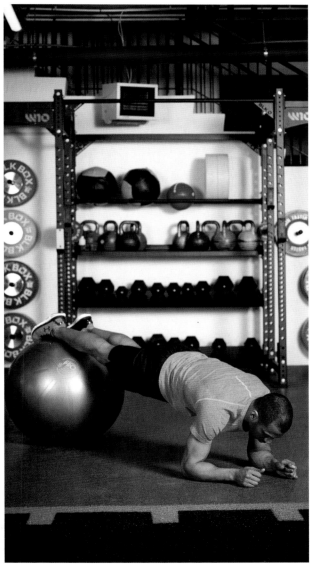

FORM Lie over a gym ball with feet flat on the floor and fingers touching your temples. Contract your abs to raise your torso up off the ball, pause at the top, then lower back to the start.

FORM Hold your body in a straight line from head to heels with your elbows directly beneath your shoulders and both feet on a gym ball. Brace your abs to hold this position without letting your hips sag.

WORKOUT 2 SHOULDERS, LEGS AND ABS

1a Cuban press

SETS 3 **REPS** 12 **TEMPO** n/a **REST** 10sec

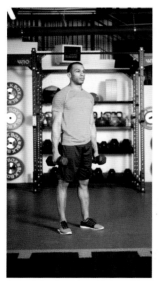
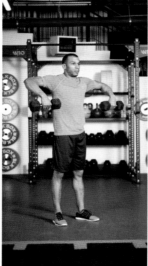
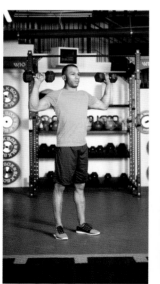
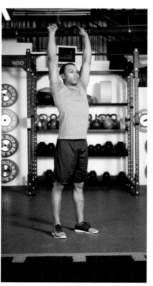

FORM Raise your arms to the sides until your elbows are bent at 90°. Keeping your upper arms horizontal, rotate your elbows until your hands point up. Press the weights directly overhead. Reverse the movement back to the start.

1b Overhead press

SETS 3 **REPS** 12 **TEMPO** 4010 **REST** 10sec

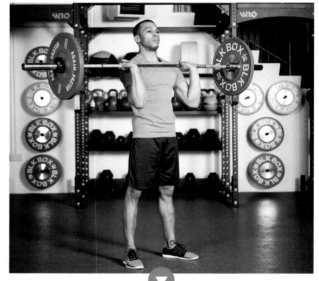
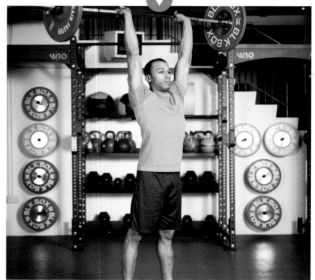

FORM Stand tall with your chest up and core braced, holding the barbell at shoulder height with palms facing forwards. Press the bar directly overhead so your arms are straight, then return slowly to the start.

1c Lateral raise

SETS 3 **REPS** 12 **TEMPO** 4010 **REST** 60sec

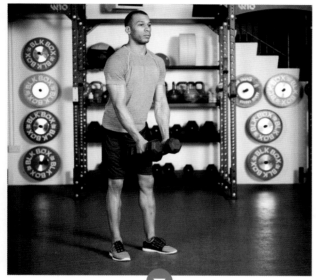

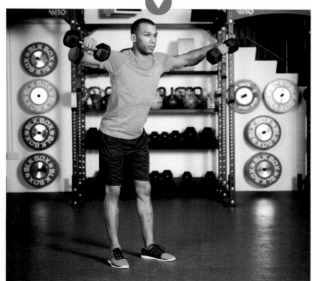

FORM Hold a light dumbbell in each hand by your sides with your palms facing one another. Keeping a slight bend in your elbows, raise the weights out to the sides making sure you use your muscles and not momentum.

2a Front squat

SETS 3 **REPS** 12 **TEMPO** 4010 **REST** 10sec

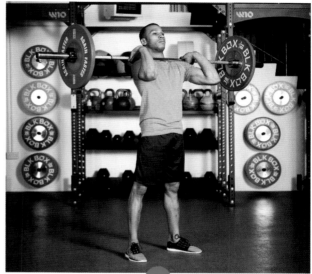

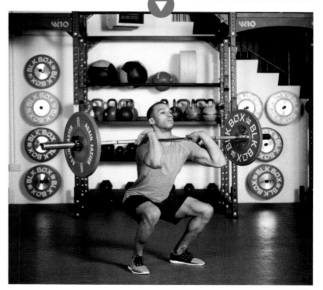

FORM Hold the bar on the front of your shoulders with your palms facing upwards. Simultaneously bend at the hips and the knees to lower towards the floor then press through your heels to stand back up again.

2b Romanian deadlift

SETS 3 **REPS** 12 **TEMPO** 4010 **REST** 10sec

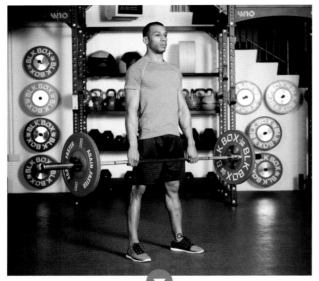

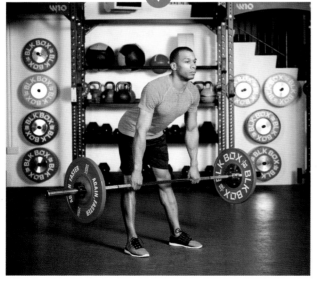

FORM Keeping a slight bend in your knees, bend forwards from the hips and lower the bar down the front of your shins until you feel a good stretch in your hamstrings. Reverse the move back to the start by pushing your hips forwards.

2c Mountain climber

SETS 3 **REPS** 12 **TEMPO** n/a **REST** 60sec

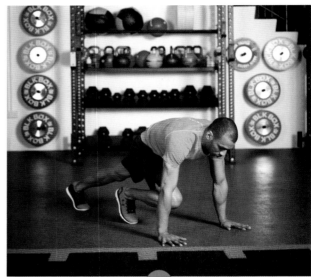

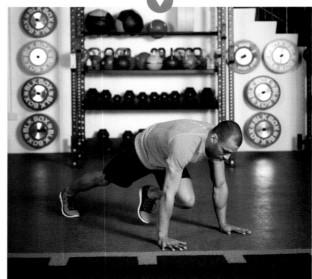

FORM Start in a position similar to a sprinter on the starting blocks. Bring one knee forwards and towards your arms, then back to the start. Repeat with the other leg, keeping the movement slow and controlled.

3a Gym ball crunch twist

SETS 3 **REPS** 12 **TEMPO** 3010 **REST** 10sec

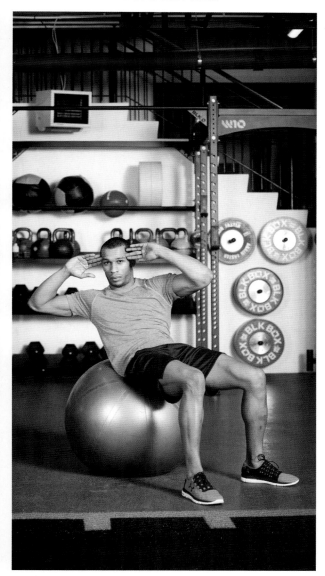

FORM Lie over a Swiss ball with feet flat on the floor and fingers touching your temples. Contract your abs to raise your torso up off the ball, then rotate to one side. Pause at the top, lower back to the start, then repeat to the other side.

3b Gym ball incline plank

SETS 3 **TIME** 40secs **REST** 60sec

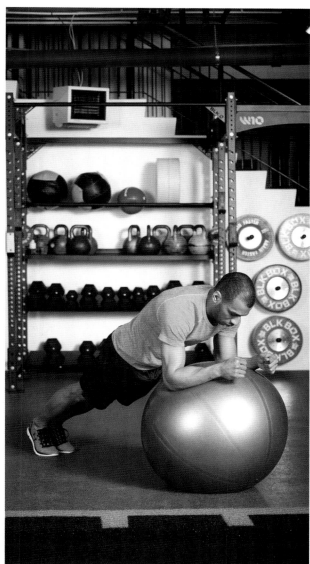

FORM Hold your body in a straight line from head to heels with your elbows on a gym ball directly beneath your shoulders. Brace your abs to hold this position without letting your hips sag.

WORKOUT 3 ARMS AND ABS

1a Incline biceps curl

SETS 3 REPS 12 TEMPO 4010 REST 10sec

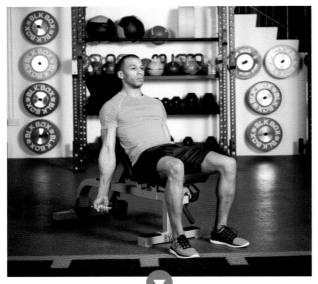

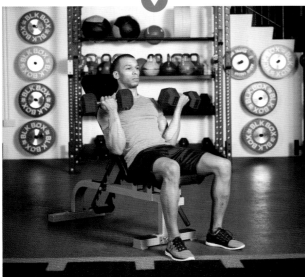

FORM Keeping your back flat against the bench and your elbows close to your sides, curl both dumbbells up to shoulder height. Squeeze your biceps at the top of the move, then slowly return the start.

1b Hammer curl

SETS 3 REPS 12 TEMPO 4010 REST 10sec

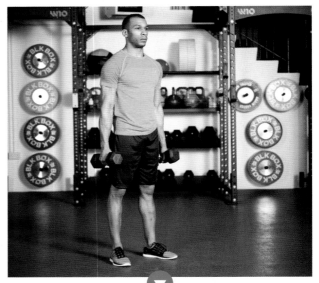

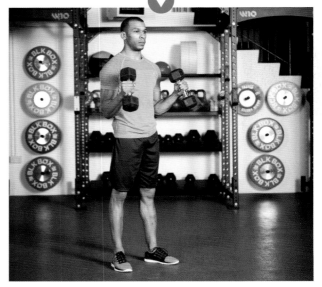

FORM With your palms facing in and your elbows tucked in to your sides, curl the dumbbells up towards your chest, squeezing your biceps at the top. Lower under control to return to the start position.

1c Alternating biceps curl

SETS 3 **REPS** 12 **TEMPO** 4010 **REST** 60sec

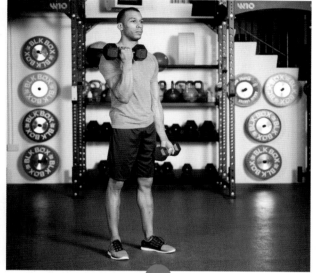

2a Lying triceps extension

SETS 3 **REPS** 12 **TEMPO** 4010 **REST** 10sec

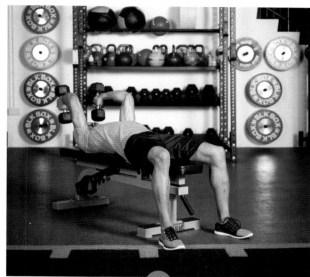

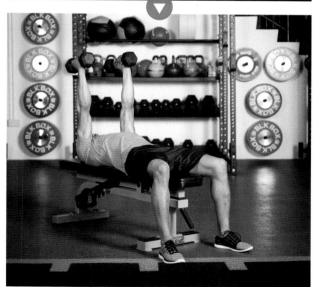

FORM Hold a pair of dumbbells with your palms facing forwards. Keeping your elbows tucked in to your sides, curl one dumbbell up towards your chest, then lower it and raise the other.

FORM Slowly lower the weights towards the top of your head by bending your elbows, keeping your upper arms as still as possible. Without arching your back, slowly return the weights to the start position by straightening your arms.

2b Bench dip

SETS 3 **REPS** 12 **TEMPO** 4010 **REST** 10sec

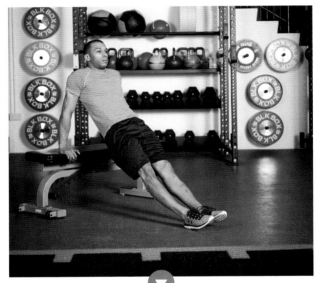

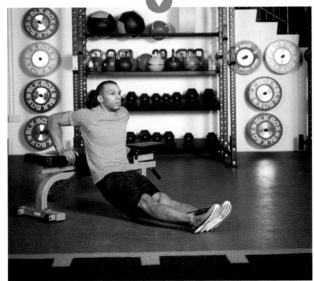

FORM Place your palms on a bench with your legs straight and out in front of you. Bend at the elbows to lower towards the floor, ensuring that your elbows don't flare outwards, then press back up to the start.

2c Eccentric diamond press-up

SETS 3 **REPS** 12 **TEMPO** 4010 **REST** 60sec

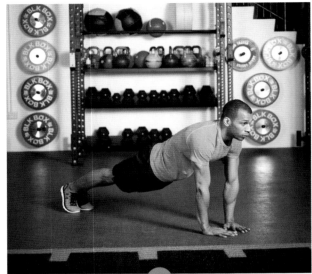

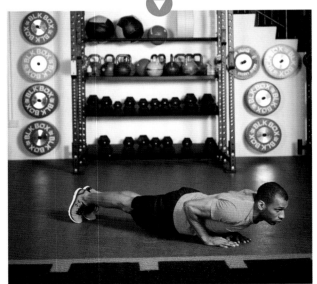

FORM Placing your hands close together so your thumbs and index fingers touch, lower your torso until your chest is just above the floor then go onto your knees to get back to the start and repeat the move.

3a Gym ball crunch

SETS 3 **REPS** 12 **TEMPO** 3010 **REST** 10sec

3b Gym ball rollout

SETS 3 **REPS** 12 **TEMPO** 4010 **REST** 60sec

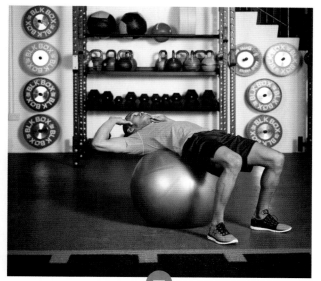

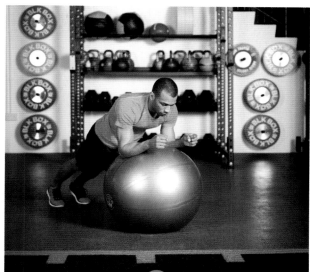

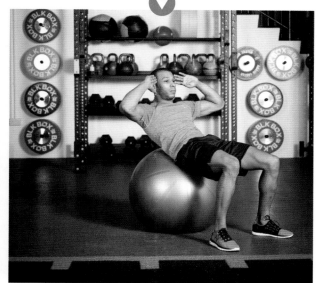

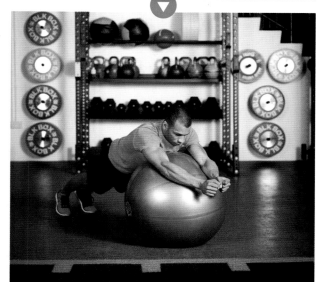

FORM Lie over a Swiss ball with feet flat on the floor and fingers touching your temples. Contract your upper abs to raise your torso up off the ball, pause at the top, then lower back to the start.

FORM Kneel in front of a Swiss ball with both elbows resting on arm. Keeping your core braced, roll the ball away from your knees until your body forms a straight line from head to hips. Pause, then reverse the movement back to the start.

Mind, Body & Soul

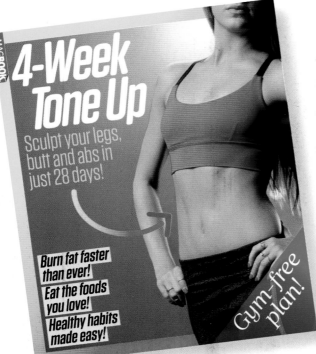
This is your essential guide to shaping and sculpting a stronger, leaner and more defined body in just 28 days. This book is split into three distinct exercise chapters – legs, butt and abs – to help you get to work fast on improving the body part you most want to target. That way you can start looking and feeling better than ever as soon as possible.

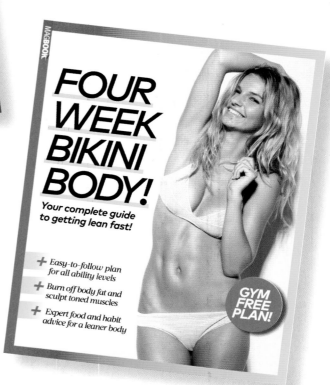
Complete guide to toning up your body in just four weeks. Following a simple step-by-step programme, you'll burn more fat and develop lean, defined muscles. Plus, learn good habits that will make you healthier for life.
Spring 2019 – Available to pre-order